A Guide to Global Mental Health Practice

T0074917

Drawing on the authors' experience in developing and implementing global mental health programs in crisis and development settings, *A Guide to Global Mental Health Practice: Seeing the Unseen* is designed for mental health, public health, and primary care professionals new to this emerging area.

The guide is organized topically and divided into four sections that move from organizing and delivering global mental health services to clinical practice, and from various settings and populations likely to be encountered to special issues unique to global work. Case studies based around a central scene are threaded throughout the book to convey what global mental health work actually involves.

Mental health professionals of all backgrounds, including social workers, nurses, nurse practitioners, psychologists, and psychiatrists, as well as public health professionals and community level medical professionals and mental health advocates will benefit from this engaging primer. It is the book for anyone committed to addressing mental health issues in a low resource or crisis-hit setting, whether international or domestic.

Craig L. Katz, M.D. is Associate Clinical Professor of Psychiatry and Medical Education at Icahn School of Medicine at Mount Sinai, New York, USA.

Jan Schuetz-Mueller, M.D. is Assistant Professor of Psychiatry at Icahn School of Medicine at Mount Sinai, New York, USA.

A Guide to Global Mental Health Practice

Seeing the Unseen

Craig L. Katz and
Jan Schuetz-Mueller
with contributions from Richard E. Fuerch,
Linda Chokroverty, and Karen Carpio Barrantes

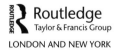
Routledge
Taylor & Francis Group

LONDON AND NEW YORK

First published 2015
by Routledge
2 Park Square, Milton Park, Abingdon, Oxon OX14 4RN

and by Routledge
711 Third Avenue, New York, NY 10017

Routledge is an imprint of the Taylor & Francis Group, an informa business

British Library Cataloguing-in-Publication Data
A catalogue record for this book is available from the British Library

Library of Congress Cataloging in Publication Data
Katz, Craig L., author.
A guide to global mental health practice : seeing the unseen / Craig L.
Katz and Jan Schuetz-Mueller.
    p. ; cm.
  Includes bibliographical references.
  I. Schuetz-Mueller, Jan, author. II. Title.
  [DNLM: 1. Mental Disorders—Case Reports. 2. Mentally Ill
  Persons—Case Reports. 3. Internationality. 4. Mental Health
  Services. 5. Psychiatry—organization & administration—Case
  Reports. WM 140]
  RA790.55
  362.19689—dc23
  2014042678

ISBN: 9781138022164 (hbk)
ISBN: 9781138022171 (pbk)
ISBN: 9781315777221 (ebk)

Typeset in Sabon
by Keystroke, Station Road, Codsall, Wolverhampton

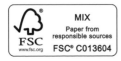

MIX
Paper from
responsible sources
FSC
www.fsc.org   FSC® C013604

Printed and bound by CPI Group (UK) Ltd, Croydon, CR0 4YY

To Linda, Maya, Lev and Sarah,
Who let us go away and make us want to come back.

Contents

Figures

Tables

Contributors and acknowledgments

Authors

Craig L. Katz, M.D.
Associate Clinical Professor of Psychiatry and Medical Education
Icahn School of Medicine at Mount Sinai
New York, NY, USA

Jan Schuetz-Mueller, M.D.
Assistant Professor of Psychiatry
Icahn School of Medicine at Mount Sinai
New York, NY, USA

Contributors

Karen Carpio Barrantes, M.P.H.
Ecole des Hautes Etudes en Santé Publique (EHESP)
Rennes, France

Linda Chokroverty, M.D., F.A.A.P.
Assistant Clinical Professor of Psychiatry and Behavioral Sciences
Assistant Clinical Professor of Pediatrics
Albert Einstein College of Medicine of Yeshiva University
Bronx, New York, USA

Richard E. Fuerch
Deputy Chief (Retired), New York City Fire Department
Long Island, New York, USA

Cover illustration

Chase Walker
www.chasewalkerart.com

Foreword

On September 11, 2001 I was on duty in the South Bronx in New York City as a Deputy Chief in the New York City Fire Department, the FDNY. The following day, I responded to what was already being called 'Ground Zero.' Along with many other firefighters, I spent the ensuing days, weeks, and months working on the rescue and recovery effort at the World Trade Center site. When we were not working at Ground Zero or working our regular tours in the firehouse, we attended countless funerals and memorial services for many of the 343 firefighters who were killed on 9/11. That experience was the beginning of a journey that brought me face to face with many of the mental health issues that exist today. Global mental health, the focus of this book, is a further extension of many of those issues.

Methods of dealing with mental health issues in today's modern world are much better than they have ever been before; however, even in our modern culture, challenges remain in recognizing, acknowledging, and treating mental health disorders.

The August 2014 suicide of actor/comedian Robin Williams presents an object lesson in the present state of mental health awareness in the United States and possibly beyond. While Mr. Williams often talked about his substance abuse problems, both alcohol and drugs, it was his publicist who, shortly after Mr. Williams's death, described him as recently suffering from 'severe depression.' To their credit, several news media outlets, both television and print, brought out experts who described 'depression' in some detail, and tried to bring the pervasiveness of this problem to the national consciousness. These news outlets also alluded to the stigma related to mental health issues, particularly with respect to 'depression.' In some reports however, depression was not even mentioned as a possible cause of the suicide. Substance abuse issues were submitted as a cause, rather than a symptom, of his illness.

Stigma, in terms of admitting mental health problems and seeking health care for these sorts of problems remains a critical factor, particularly among populations that include the military and first responders. As Dr. Katz and Dr. Schuetz-Mueller describe in Chapter 13 of this book, the issue of stigma can be even worse in the global arena in which they work. Cultural factors provide an additional challenge when dealing with mental health issues in different countries where there is widespread misunderstanding of the entire issue of mental health.

With that being said, organizations like the FDNY have met many of the challenges head on. The FDNY 'Counseling Services Unit' has existed for decades. For years, it was mainly the place to which firefighters were sent when they had to deal with alcohol and drug related problems; however, even before 9/11/2001, the Counseling Services Unit began to recognize the need to address traumatic events, such as tragic line of duty deaths, with the firefighters who were directly involved.

In February 2002, along with about one hundred firefighters, I was assigned to work exclusively in the recovery effort at the World Trade Center site. Human remains were recovered on a daily basis. It was grueling and exhausting work, both physically and emotionally. At the conclusion of this assignment, on March 1, the entire detail was gathered together for a debriefing. We were told that counseling was available for those who felt they needed it. Of course, being tough firefighters, we all said we did not need any counseling. But after returning to regular firehouse duty, I realized that something was not right with me—anger, hyper vigilance, anxiety, difficulty sleeping, and physical exhaustion were among the symptoms I experienced. I sought out the services of the FDNY counseling unit and they assisted me in dealing with those issues.

The FDNY is a unique community. Being able to commiserate around the kitchen table in the firehouse can be a form of group therapy for firefighters. The firehouse and the fire company also provide a sense of place which is so important as a form of self identification during traumatic times. It is this sense of place that is often lost among populations that are 'displaced' or 'placed,' as described in this book. The firehouse, as a secondary home, can 'hold great psychological meaning in the experience of one's self.'

I was privileged to be part of a group, including others who had a direct connection with 9/11, that accompanied Dr. Katz on two of his many trips to Japan. Along with the International Rotary Club, the Japan Medical Society, the Icahn School of Medicine at Mount Sinai, and several other organizations, the 9/11 Tribute Center helped organize several 'Good Will' visits to Japan to connect 9/11 survivors with those who suffered from the 3/11/11 Great East Japan Earthquake that spawned a tsunami and nuclear power plant disaster. The trip included attendance at a Fukushima Medical University Seminar, school visits, numerous visits to mental health clinics, as well as interactions with residents at temporary housing settlements. We also visited some of the villages decimated by the '3/11' disaster where we witnessed the damage and saw the progress being made in recovery. We interacted and shared stories with many of the survivors. By telling them our stories of dealing with the effects of 9/11 and by listening to and empathizing with their stories, I believe we contributed to their recovery.

Becoming familiar with the culture of those with whom we collaborated was a valuable part of our trip. We included visits to Buddhist Temples and Shinto Shrines. These were much more than tourist destinations, as they allowed us to become familiar with Japanese culture and thereby enabled us to better connect with our hosts. Visits with government officials and interactions with various media connections also helped spread the message of our symbolic mission.

Dr. Katz is a co-founder and former supervising psychiatrist of the World Trade Center Worker/Volunteer Mental Health Monitoring and Treatment Program for the Mount Sinai WTC Medical Monitoring Program. It has been his challenge to monitor mental health issues for a vast population of first responders, rescue and recovery workers (including emergency responders, construction workers, and volunteers) who operated at the World Trade Center on September 11, 2001, and on the days, weeks, and months following those tragic terrorist attacks. I have witnessed Dr. Katz's dedication to studying, understanding, and dealing with issues surrounding a variety of mental health issues that have arisen as a result of 3/11. As I listened to his lectures, and attended a two-day seminar at Fukushima Medical University, I came to understand his focus on not just that disaster, but on mental health issues that could arise anywhere, anytime, and under any circumstance.

Dr. Schuetz-Mueller has a varied and interesting background, having lived in Fiji, Afghanistan, and attended medical school in Vienna, Austria. With Dr. Katz, he co-directs the Mount Sinai Program in Global Mental Health, giving him a rare opportunity to explore the many facets of global mental health and to hone the perspective that he shares in this volume.

In 'Seeing the Unseen . . .' Drs. Katz and Schuetz-Mueller have provided road maps for the implementation of global mental health initiatives in worldwide environments that will be unfamiliar to most practitioners. The readability of this book signifies its focus on providing a collaborative experience with the reader, rather than simply providing information. This reflects the emphasis on collaboration that global mental health professionals must engage in when dealing with their hosts. When the groups of docents from the 9/11 Tribute Center visited Japan to empathize with the victims of 3/11, we felt that we were acting as 'Good-Will Ambassadors.' It is now apparent to me that we were also fulfilling a role as symbolic global mental health collaborators. As described in this book, collaboration is one of the keys to any successful global mental health initiative.

Richard E. Fuerch
Deputy Chief (Retired), New York City Fire Department
Long Island, New York, U.S.A.
15 September 2014

Introduction
Seeing the unseen

What follows will serve as a tour of what lies beneath the surface of things in the hearts and minds of people across the globe as they live their lives. In the vastness of human experience, we have chosen to look beneath the surface because one thing people can do that perhaps no other living thing can do, or do so well, is hide things. We especially hide our intentions and feelings. It is truly the case that with human beings, as a species and as individuals, there is always more than meets the eye. Were it otherwise, we would surely not be human as we know it.

People tend to hide those aspects of themselves about which they feel shame or guilt. They of course protect and conceal their worldly possessions out of concern for the envy and even thievery of others. But, in the emotional realm the things about which an individual feels shame or guilt are things which they believe others not only do not want but even shun. Or, if others 'possess' the knowledge of this aspect of them, that they would misuse it for their own cruel gain or gratification. Consider this account of shame and guilt (Morrison 1983):

> Shame . . . is about the whole self, and its failure to live up to an ideal; as such, it is a 'narcissistic' reaction. A typical defense against shame is hiding, or running away . . . Guilt, on the other hand, refers to a transgression, an action, and therefore has a more specific cognitive or behavioral antecedent than shame, referring less globally to the subjective sense of self . . . Shame . . . results from incapacity. Guilt for transgression.

Shame in particular has been described as a broad spectrum of painful emotions, including embarrassment, humiliation, mortification, and disgrace, that accompany the feeling of being rejected, ridiculed, exposed, or of losing the respect of others (Tuckett & Levinson 2010).

We want to focus on those aspects of their inner selves about which people feel shame. And, really, then we wish to address the loneliness that people feel in the world around them because of their fears, realistic or otherwise, about how they might be viewed by others 'if only they knew' that they felt a certain way, desired certain things, or perceived in potentially unique ways. If an individual experiences psychological pain, his or her isolation can surely be protective in some settings and with some people. But, if misplaced or overdone, isolation only compounds psychological suffering. This is captured in the 1883 poem by Ella Wheeler Wilcox, *Solitude*:

Laugh, and the world laughs with you;
Weep and you weep alone.
For the sad old earth must borrow its mirth,
But has trouble enough of its own.
Sing, and the hills will answer;
Sigh, it is lost on the air.
The echoes bound to a joyful sound,
But shrink from voicing care.
   Rejoice, and men will seek you;
Grieve, and they turn and go.
They want full measure of all your pleasure,
But they do not need your woe.
Be glad, and your friends are many;
Be sad, and you lose them all.
There are none to decline your nectared wine,
But alone you must drink life's gall.
   Feast, and your halls are crowded;
Fast, and the world goes by.
Succeed and give, and it helps you live,
But no man can help you die.
There is room in the halls of pleasure
For a long and lordly train,
But one by one we must all file on
Through the narrow aisles of pain.

Born in Wisconsin and later moving to New York and finally Connecticut, Mrs. Wheeler Wilcox was of course American from cradle to grave, and the pathos of her poem could well reflect the vastness she found growing up in the heartland of America. Our tour of the unseen makes an assumption that her wish for the company of others in good times and in bad is one that is universal and cross-cultural. Most everyone needs the acceptance and ministrations of others when things are bad. And, most people want this, too. If they do not, this probably says more about them as individuals then about their cultures. We have not yet encountered a culture or society that inherently and unswervingly shuns the sharing of either good or bad emotions, even if there are variations in how they do this.

   Importantly, human beings also have the capacity to conceal how they feel and think even from themselves. Freud famously elucidated models of the mind that involved an unconscious and described a form of human suffering related to it. Here, desirous or aggressive feelings that are too uncomfortable for an individual are, unbeknownst to them, 'suppressed' by their mind into a portion of itself of which they are not aware. The different mechanisms the mind employs to accomplish this can lead to unhealthy (i.e., kicking the family dog when one was angry at one's boss) or healthy (i.e., instead going for a much needed jog upon arriving home) results. The tour in this book therefore involves to some degree a looking inward into ourselves as much as others.

Mental health

In referencing the emotional life of people, our aspiration as psychiatrists is to help people everywhere to lead the most emotionally healthy lives they can. And, so at the center of our focus lies mental health, which simply is not possible if people feel too alone or too shunned, whether or not they have a 'diagnosable' mental illness. The latter we will discuss in later chapters, especially Chapter 1 on the epidemiology of mental illness, but here we want to be clear about what we mean by mental health. It is not easily defined and is more readily described. But, one reasonable working definition of mental health is as follows: a state of balance among the internal forces in one's life as well as between the internal forces and the external forces that are brought to bear (Wallace 1983). Even more to the point is the definition of mental health given by one student of ours—*emotional wellbeing*.

A psychiatric researcher, Dr. George Vaillant, has taken these definitions even further and offered an essentially holistic view on the matter. He has espoused the idea that there are seven different ways to define mental health and that, in fact, there is evidence to believe that they are all different facets of the same things, as follows: exceeding a score on scale or survey of mental health; having multiple human strengths and few weaknesses; maturity; positive emotions; high socio-emotional intelligence; subjective wellbeing; and resilience (Vaillant 2012). Just as important for the globally oriented health professional, he uses the analogy of a decathlete to explain how to grapple with this list of definitions:

> A decathlon star must possess muscle strength, speed, endurance, grace and competitive grit, although the combinations may vary. Amongst decathlon champions, the general definition will not differ from nation to nation, or century to century. The salience of a given facet of a decathlon champion, or of mental health, may vary from culture to culture, but all facets are important.

Global mental health needs

A focus on the mental health of the world is further necessitated by a reality that goes beyond how individuals grapple with their own experiences and suffering to how they grapple with that of others.

As will be laid out in detail in later chapters, societies do not tend to prioritize mental health issues. Governments tend not to fund mental health services adequately, if at all. What occurs is a conspiracy of silence around mental health issues. Maybe the position of shame, loneliness, and inattention with which many people around the world greet their own inner life and mental health jeopardizes the likelihood that they will be any kinder to others.

It should not be surprising to find appalling statistics regarding the extent of untreated mental illness around the world. An illustrative 2002–2003 survey of 60,463 adults in 14 countries estimated that in the 6 less developed countries in the study (China, Colombia, Lebanon, Mexico, Nigeria, and Ukraine), 76.3–85.4 percent of individuals with what they defined as severe cases of mental illness did not receive any treatment in the 12 months preceding the study (Demyttenaere et al. 2004). This encompassed individuals with either bipolar disorder ('manic-depression') or a severe alcohol use disorder or who either had made a suicide attempt or suffered severe impairment in function or distress level in association with any of the psychiatric diagnoses. And, even in the more developed countries (Belgium, France, Germany, Italy, Netherlands, Spain, United States, Japan), 35.5 to 50.3 percent of these same classes of individuals were estimated to have gone without treatment over that same period (including 47.7 percent in the United States).

These results should humble us for three reasons. First, there is no reason to think they are not generalizable to other countries in the world. Second, as these figures only focus on cases of a great severity, the numbers would indeed worsen if mental health conditions of all severity were considered. This is consistent with experience since in countries where there are scarce resources for mental health care, typically only the sickest of the sick receive attention. Even in high income countries, the mild to moderately mentally ill population receives less care than the most severely ill. For example, in the United States, 34.1 percent and 22.5 percent, respectively, of people with moderate and mild mental health problems received care. Third, even though the study also indicates that higher income countries do a better job of providing mental health treatment than lower income countries, their efforts can still overlook up to half of the severely mentally ill.

On the last point, policymakers if not the average citizen often charge that mental health care is a luxury relative to other health needs, let alone other needs. So, even if we classify so many people in so many places as having untreated mental illness of some severity, the matter could then be dismissed as lacking relevance to the public's health. Typically, those with mental health problems are dichotomized into two extremes that somehow both seem to absolve society of responsibility—the severely ill and the mildly ill. The usual societal response to the former is to deposit the most mentally ill in old style 'mental asylums' where they are given up on and warehoused out of sight and out of mind, at least in the developing world (Rudolf 2013). As for the latter view, news stories too numerous to cite repeatedly argue that psychiatry has become an industry where the 'worried well' receive too much attention and psychiatrists too much profit.

However, statistics about the impact of mental health problems on functioning (or morbidity) belie any grounds for labeling them a luxury that society cannot afford. Major Depression is the second leading cause of disability worldwide and is in the top four of such causes in every single one of the six global regions in the 2010 Global Burden of Disease Study (Whiteford et al. 2013). And, when taken together, the category of mental health disorders constitutes a larger cause of morbidity than any other category, including cardiovascular diseases and cancers. This state of affairs has led to the following lament from experts: 'According to virtually any metric, grave concern is warranted with regard to the high global burden of mental disorders, the associated intransigent, unmet needs, and the unacceptable toll of human suffering' (Becker & Kleinman 2013).

Defining global mental health

Global health has been defined as:

> an area for study, research, and practice that places a priority on improving health and achieving equity in health for all people worldwide. Global health emphasizes

transnational health issues, determinants, and solutions; involves many disciplines within and beyond the health sciences and promotes interdisciplinary collaboration; and is a synthesis of population based prevention with individual-level clinical care.

(Koplan et al. 2009)

We therefore can define global mental health as this definition applied to mental health (Patel & Prince 2010).

In practice, global mental health, like global health, aspires to work on behalf of both the individual and the public's mental health, ambitiously taking on clinical and society-level needs. However, in this book, we take a stance that encourages a more public health oriented approach to mental health for at least two reasons. We believe that Western psychiatry has been too focused on the ill patient and not enough on the healthy one, prioritizing mental illness and disorder over mental health. A public health/prevention slanted stance around mental health is one a country of any income level can benefit from. Hence, global mental health from this perspective reflects a truly global practice and not simply one in which the mental health 'haves' give to the 'have not's.'

There is a second very pragmatic reason for adopting a public health approach to global mental health needs, and that is the extent to which they are ignored. There are just too many people with too many overlooked mental health problems in too many places in the world to enable a mental health practitioner from the 'haves' to be able to make a sufficient enough impact on the world by providing direct care in a far off land. Psychiatry involves long-term care of a usually pharmacologic and/or psycho-therapeutic nature and long-term relationships on the order of months to years— most practicing mental health professionals cannot possibly provide these in both their home community and in the needy community of interest to them.

So, in this book, when we talk about global mental health 'practice' we are not referring to clinical practice and are not necessarily encouraging mental health professionals to open up clinical practices in underserved areas of their country or the world. By global mental health practice, we mean *collaborative activities conducted by health, mental health, and allied health professionals and community and government partners which improve access to mental health care and maintenance for all people in all places.* Given the multi-disciplinary nature of this practice, throughout the book we will refer to those working in the field of global mental health variously as global mental health practitioners, professionals, workers, contributors, and, where appropriate, clinicians, students, and researchers.

In their comprehensive definition of global health, Koplan et al. (2009) reference global health study and research in addition to practice. This book is premised on the expectation that study is a prerequisite for going into an unfamiliar community or country to work in global mental health. Preparation and learning position the global mental health professional to maximize their impact and to ensure that they give at least as much as they get. As for research, we follow the excellent discussion by Tol et al. (2012) that contrasts the differing values of academic excellence among researchers and practical relevance among workers in the humanitarian aid setting while finding common ground for the good of global mental health. They discuss what can be called 'implementation science' or science that somehow bridges the practical needs of service delivery in global mental health and the demands of academic rigor. Their message for the global mental health practitioner is ours—if you are provided with adequate training and resources, it is possible to integrate research into your practice.

To this we add that the scarcity of psychiatric research outside of high income countries creates an imperative to research, write, and publish among health, mental health, and allied health professionals. An analysis of research trials on psychiatric treatments in fact has revealed that 86.8 percent of them were conducted in high income countries, 12.3 percent in middle income countries, and 0.9 percent in low income countries (Patel et al. 2007). In conducting research about their interventions, global mental health professionals help not only to assure the quality of their efforts and justify funding outlays by funders but also to archive the nature of the work and its strengths and weaknesses for future global mental health workers and efforts. It becomes another way to multiply the efforts of global mental health professionals beyond the clinical encounter.

This book

It should be apparent by now that global mental health practitioners have an enormous amount of issues to learn and to address. The needs are high and the expectations for how to address them in an impactful way are higher. And, again, much of their work must go on among people, things, and issues that are too often unseen and felt to be best left that way. For the practitioner who plans to work in a community or country far from home and their usual way of life and practice, the personal dimensions of the work only add layers to the challenges.

The book chapters progress through the topics we believe to be most helpful for global mental health practice, providing at least a survival guide and ideally a guide for thriving in the work and its fruits. The first part talks about systems level issues fundamental to the practice of global mental health. Chapter 1 begins with the epidemiology of worldwide mental health problems, laying out the scope of the needs from a disease perspective. Chapters 2 and 3 then draw a picture of the non-human and human resources typically available and necessary to meet this need. Chapter 4 addresses an issue that global mental health professionals find especially daunting, that of how conditions of scarcity or poverty interact with mental wellbeing.

The next part addresses clinical issues. Chapter 5 expands on the issues around medications and mental health touched upon in Chapter 2 whereas Chapter 6 expands on the topic of human resources from Chapter 3 by exploring the use of psychotherapy and psychotherapists around the world. Chapter 7 then rounds out the discussion of clinical interventions by discussing the use of complementary and alternative treatments in various parts of the world with a special emphasis on the role of healers.

What follow are chapters on special populations. Chapter 8 by Linda Chokroverty focuses on children and adolescents, Chapter 9 looks at issues unique to disaster affected communities, Chapter 10 defines and addresses displaced, or 'placed,' populations, and Chapter 11 examines issues in rural psychiatry.

Finally the last part examines special issues. Chapter 12 reviews the history of misuse of psychiatry by governments and other entities, while Chapter 13 delves into the inexorable stigma surrounding mental illness and its care. Chapter 14 discusses an overall framework within which to practice global mental health known as the 'Wheel of Global Mental Health.' Finally, Chapter 15 prescribes the personal preparations for global mental health work. The book culminates with an Appendix written by Karen Carpio Barrantes that integrates the key ideas of all fifteen chapters into an algorithm for 'scaling up' mental health services in low resource settings.

The platform

The book takes as its starting point a photo conjured from the experiences and photo albums of the authors. Imagined to be a photo from the front page of a Western newspaper, it wraps around the cover of this book and also follows this chapter, depicting a group of people going about their lives on a dry but vibrant street. The scene rests on a caption that reads, 'People return to the streets after leaving behind the battleground' below which lies the story of a far off low income country staggering to its feet after a truce in a brutal 5-year long civil war.

It is a photo and story not unfamiliar to many Western consumers of news and for good reason. According to ReliefWeb (http://reliefweb.int/countries), they are monitoring 68 crises and disasters around the world even as this Introduction is being written on December 15, 2014. Meanwhile, they monitored 115 such events in the last full calendar year of 2013 and in the last ten years saw a peak of 195 in 2009.

In what follows, each chapter will begin with a vignette highlighting a person from the photo that illuminates their life outside of the frame of the photo. The reader will find how each of their lives somehow touches on something in the field of global mental health specific to the topic(s) in that chapter. Even some of the objects in the photo will prove relevant as well. Where appropriate the chapters will return to the storyline.

So, we have referred to the book as a tour, a guide, and a story. In all, we hope the newspaper image and the people's lives beyond it make it a hands-on tour and make the learning experience an immersive one. And, through it all may the reader come to better see the unseen and help others to do the same.

References

Becker, A.E. & Kleinman, A. 2013, 'Mental health and the global agenda,' *The New England Journal of Medicine,* vol. 369, no. 14, pp. 1380–1381.

Demyttenaere, K., Bruffaerts, R., Posada-Villa, J., Gasquet, I., Kovess, V., Lepine, J.P., Angermeyer, M.C., Bernert, S., de Girolamo, G., & Morosini, P. 2004, 'Prevalence, severity, and unmet need for treatment of mental disorders in the World Health Organization World Mental Health Surveys,' *JAMA: The Journal of the American Medical Association,* vol. 291, no. 21, pp. 2581–2590.

Koplan, J.P., Bond, T.C., Merson, M.H., Reddy, K.S., Rodriguez, M.H., Sewankambo, N.K., & Wasserheit, J.N. 2009, 'Towards a common definition of global health,' *The Lancet,* vol. 373, no. 9679, pp. 1993–1995.

Morrison, A.P. 1983, 'Shame, ideal self, and narcissism,' *Contemporary Psychoanalysis,* vol. 19, pp. 295–318.

Patel, V. & Prince, M. 2010, 'Global mental health: a new global health field comes of age,' *JAMA: The Journal of the American Medical Association,* vol. 303, no. 19, pp. 1976–1977.

Patel, V., Araya, R., Chatterjee, S., Chisholm, D., Cohen, A., De Silva, M., Hosman, C., McGuire, H., Rojas, G., & van Ommeren, M. 2007, 'Treatment and prevention of mental disorders in low-income and middle-income countries,' *The Lancet,* vol. 370, no. 9591, pp. 991–1005.

Rudolf, J. 2013, 'Where mental asylums live on'. Available: www.nytimes.com/2013/11/03/opinion/sunday/where-mental-asylums-live-on.html?pagewanted=all (accessed September 17, 2014).

Tol, W.A., Patel, V., Tomlinson, M., Baingana, F., Galappatti, A., Silove, D., Sondorp, E., van Ommeren, M., Wessells, M.G., & Panter-Brick, C. 2012, 'Relevance or excellence? Setting research priorities for mental health and psychosocial support in humanitarian settings,' *Harvard Review of Psychiatry,* vol. 20, no. 1, pp. 25–36.

Tuckett, D. & Levinson, N.A. 2010, *PEP Consolidated Psychoanalytic Glossary,* Psychoanalytic Electronic Publishing, Delaware.

Vaillant, G.E. 2012, 'Positive mental health: is there a cross-cultural definition?,' *World Psychiatry: Official Journal of the World Psychiatric Association (WPA),* vol. 11, no. 2, pp. 93–99.

Wallace, E. 1983, *Dynamic Psychiatry in Theory and Practice,* Lea and Febiger, Michigan.

Wheeler Wilcox, E. 1883, *Solitude.* Available: http://en.wikipedia.org/wiki/Solitude_(poem) (accessed January 19, 2014).

Whiteford, H.A., Degenhardt, L., Rehm, J., Baxter, A.J., Ferrari, A.J., Erskine, H.E., Charlson, F.J., Norman, R.E., Flaxman, A.D., & Johns, N. 2013, 'Global burden of disease attributable to mental and substance use disorders: findings from the Global Burden of Disease Study 2010,' *The Lancet,* vol. 382, no. 9904, pp. 1575–1586.

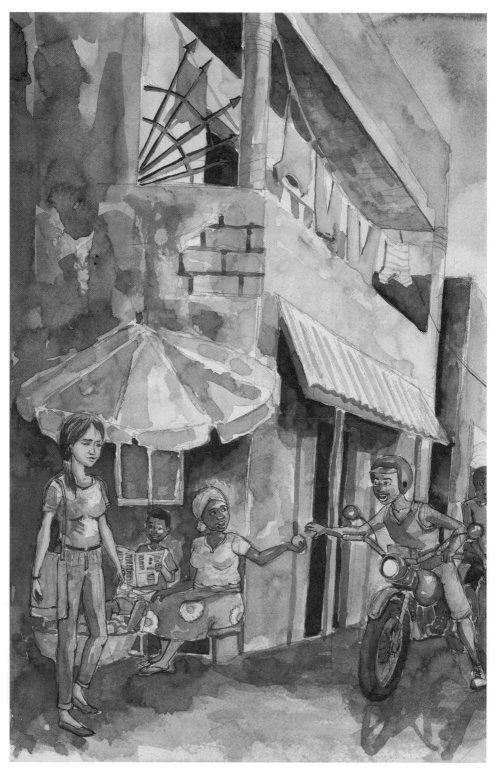

People return to the streets after leaving behind the battleground.

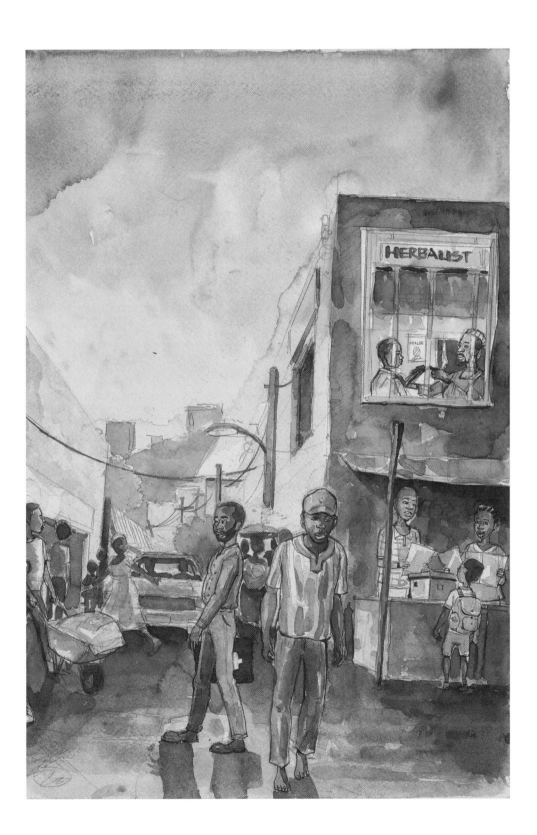

Part I

Organizing for global mental health

Chapter 1

Epidemiology

Sam walks languidly among the hustle and bustle of the street. He is a farmer who on most any other day other than his church-going Sundays would be out at this hour tending to his rice crops. Today he has left the farm in the hands of his younger brother in order to go see the doctor.

Sam has been feeling tired like never before. He's also been losing weight like it was his to spare. He fears he has malaria, a disease he lost a much younger sister to several years before. For many in his village, they deal with malaria like it were a passing headache, but he cannot shake it. He wonders if the family has been cursed.

Sam's farm survived the civil war but barely. Early on he saved most of his land from a fire ignited by nearby carpet-bombing of a warlord, only to have guerillas torch his equipment shed on their march to peace talks. The typhoon soon brought rains that were too much, too late and biblical enough to drown his nascent crops but end the war. When peace came, many of his buyers had just disappeared.

It has been a struggle for Sam and his family, making his lassitude incomprehensible. His great shame for letting his family down fueled today's three-hour bus ride into the capital city to visit the hospital. The photo captures Sam in mid stroll towards the hospital gates after he disembarked at the central bus stop in the city.

Fatigue can have myriad causes from the non-medical to both physical and psychiatric diagnoses. The medical concept of differential diagnosis captures the framework for identifying the range of likely explanations for someone's symptom(s). The capable clinician uses their training and acumen to narrow down the possibilities through history taking, physical examination and, where possible, laboratory and other testing. In this chapter, we will discuss the range of possible diagnoses that could explain Sam's problem by examining population level data about health and mental health conditions as well as experience from the field.

General health considerations

Historically when both health professionals and even the lay public in the developed world thought about the health needs of the developing world, infectious or so-called communicable diseases came to mind. This perception and reality became enshrined in global health policy with the promulgation of the Millennium Development Goals (MDG) in 2000 (United Nations 2014; Sachs & McArthur 2005). The MDG set out eight goals for addressing extreme poverty at the dawn of the new millennium.

The eight goals to have been met by 2015 are as follows: eradicating extreme poverty and hunger; achieving universal primary education; promoting gender equality and empowering women; reducing child mortality; improving maternal health; ensuring environmental sustainability; global partnership for development; and, notably, combatting HIV/AIDS, malaria, and other infectious diseases.

Depending upon where we situate his low income country, Sam has good reason for concern about malaria, if not other communicable diseases. According to the WHO, 3.3 billion people worldwide were at risk for contracting malaria in 2011 despite impressive gains made towards eradicating it as part of the MDG (World Health Organization 2014a). Worldwide efforts have made a difference with the other communicable diseases as well, but still there is reason for great concern. In 2012, 8.6 million people worldwide acquired tuberculosis (TB), with over a million dying from it even though the incidence and mortality from TB has been declining (World Health Organization 2014b). Meanwhile, 34 million people were living with HIV/AIDS in 2011, with regions such as sub-Saharan Africa representing a disproportionate portion of the global burden. In that year, 1 in 20 adults in that region had HIV/AIDS (World Health Organization 2014c). Finally, varying gains have been made among the neglected tropical diseases such as schistosomiasis and leprosy (World Health Organization 2014c).

But, there are increasingly concerns about non-infectious diseases around the world. Notably absent from the MDG were chronic medical conditions, otherwise known as non-communicable disease (NCD) (Beaglehole et al. 2007). These include in particular cardiovascular disease (high blood pressure, heart disease, and stroke), chronic respiratory conditions (asthma, emphysema, and related conditions), cancer, and diabetes. At around the time when the world was embarking on its pursuit of the MDG, communicable diseases accounted for around 32 percent of worldwide mortality whereas NCD actually accounted for 59 percent. NCD accounted for 87 percent of deaths in high income countries but also for 54 percent of deaths in low and middle income countries (Magnusson 2009). Importantly, unlike with communicable diseases, studies have shown that basic public health oriented preventative measures such as tobacco cessation and dietary salt reduction can have an impressive impact. Yet, the feeling is that NCD and the highly non-technical solutions to them have not been adequately embraced and prioritized by the WHO (Beaglehole et al. 2007).

From a statistical point of view Sam could be right that he had malaria, and any doctor in an endemic area would be remiss not to consider it as a possible explanation for his fatigue. They likewise might consider TB, neglected tropical diseases, and HIV/AIDS. But, there are increasingly other less dramatic and more insidious possible explanations. Fatigue is a common presentation for new onset diabetes, although typically with other complaints such as intense thirst or frequent urination that his doctor could explore with him. Or, depending upon his age and lifestyle factors such as diet and substance use, Sam could be developing heart disease. If he smoked, he could be developing significant respiratory problems such as emphysema.

Mental health considerations

What about Sam's mental health? The 2010 Global Burden of Disease, Injuries, and Risk Factors Study (GBD) provides the most comprehensive picture to date of worldwide mortality and morbidity from health as well as mental health conditions (Whiteford et al. 2013). It provides an invaluable perspective on the presence that mental illness has around the world and therefore requires some explaining. Three specific measures were looked at by the GBD investigators, as follows: (1) Years of Life Lost (YLL), which is a measure of premature mortality; (2) Years Lived with Disability (YLD), which is a measure of morbidity; and (3) Disability Adjusted Life Years (DALY), which results from summing YLL and YLD. DALY represents a composite view of the years of life lost to premature death or disability.

As seen in Table 1.1, mental and substance use disorders (they are grouped together) account for only 0.5 percent of worldwide mortality or YLL. Given that problems with mental health more commonly affect quality of life and functioning in daily life rather than threatening life itself, this makes sense. Instead and consistent with what was discussed earlier, four categories account for much of worldwide mortality: cardiovascular disease, cancer, infectious diseases, and neonatal conditions. Conversely, when morbidity or YLD are examined, mental and substance use disorders account for 22.9 percent of global YLD and therefore as a category constitute the number one cause of morbidity. Musculoskeletal disorders are a close second at 21.3 percent, followed by NCD at 11.1 percent. When mortality and morbidity are then examined together in worldwide DALY, mental and substance use disorders are fifth among all

Table 1.1 Proportion of YLD, YLL, and DALY explained by the ten leading causes of total burden in 2010

	Proportion of total DALY (95% UI)	Proportion of total YLD (95% UI)	Proportion of total YLL (95% UI)
Cardiovascular and circulatory diseases	11·9% (11·0–12·6)	2·8% (2·4–3·4)	15·9% (15·0–16·8)
Diarrhoea, lower respiratory infections, meningitis, and other common infectious diseases	11·4% (10·3–12·7)	2·6% (2·0–3·2)	15·4% (14·0–17·1)
Neonatal disorders	8·1% (7·3–9·0)	1·2% (1·0–1·5)	11·2% (10·2–12·4)
Cancer	7·6% (7·0–8·2)	0·6% (0·5–0·7)	10·7% (10·0–11·4)
Mental and substance use disorders	7·4% (6·2–8·6)	22·9% (18·6–27·2)	0·5% (0·4–0·7)
Musculoskeletal disorders	6·8% (5·4–8·2)	21·3% (17·7–24·9)	0·2% (0·2–0·3)
HIV/AIDS and tuberculosis	5·3% (4·8–5·7)	1·4% (1·0–1·9)	7·0% (6·4–7·5)
Other non-communicable diseases	5·1% (4·1–6·6)	11·1% (8·2–15·2)	2·4% (2·0–2·8)
Diabetes, urogenital, blood, and endocrine diseases	4·9% (4·4–5·5)	7·3% (6·1–8·7)	3·8% (3·4–4·3)
Unintentional injuries other than transport injuries	4·8% (4·4–5·3)	3·4% (2·5–4·4)	5·5% (4·9–5·9)

Source: Reproduced with permission from Whiteford et al. 2013

causes, following right behind the same top four causes of YLL that were just described (Whiteford et al. 2013).

When all measures are considered, mental and substance use disorders account for 14 percent of the total global burden of disease and are expected to climb to 15 percent by 2020 (Ngui et al. 2010). For Sam, we do not know whether he suffers from a potentially life threatening condition, whether infectious or otherwise. But, we do know that he is concerned about how poorly he has been functioning recently in his work as a farmer. And, so, given its place among disabling conditions in the world's population, mental and substance use disorders should really be a consideration as one possible explanation for Sam's lassitude. Now let's examine what we know about the worldwide scope of the specific mental disorders in order to hone our consideration of mental health reasons for his coming to the doctor.

Depressive disorders

The depressive disorders, or what might be called clinical depression, consist of Major Depression, a typically more intense and episodic mood problem, and Dysthymia, which is by definition more persistent but less intense. Both entail a fundamental complaint involving low mood or loss of pleasure in things but, as syndromes, they also involve a potential range of changes in how people think, act, or feel physically. These encompass disturbances in sleep, appetite, energy level, mental or motor speed, concentration, and self-confidence. At the most extreme, Major Depression can also involve suicide or even psychotic perceptions or thinking (American Psychiatric Association 2013).

In the 2010 Global Burden of Disease study, Major Depression in particular was found to be number two worldwide among all disorders as a cause of years lost to disability. The leading cause was low back pain. Dysthymia was only 19th. In some regions of the world, Major Depression was the leading cause of YLD, including Latin America, Southeast Asia, and Oceania whereas it was otherwise largely second in most other regions, including North America. In DALY, Major Depression was 11th among all causes, and Dysthymia was 51st, as they were not directly associated with any significant mortality. Major Depression was also found to be a contributor to the DALY-based global burden from suicide and, perhaps more surprisingly, heart disease (Ferrari et al. 2013a).

When Major Depression is looked at through the prism of its prevalence, some investigators have found that its overall worldwide point prevalence amounts to 4.7 percent across all available studies in the published literature (Ferrari et al. 2013b). If accurate, this would mean that 4.7 percent of the world's population suffers from Major Depression at any one time. Researchers also appear to agree that Major Depression is prevalent across all regions of the world, although potentially more frequently occurring in high income countries but more persistent in low and middle income countries (and hence potentially equally prevalent over any one year) (Bromet et al. 2011).

Despite its singular impact on worldwide morbidity, Major Depression is rarely the focus of much clinical attention in low and middle income countries and other low resource settings. We do not have an evidence-based explanation for this disparity, but surmise that the fact of depression's being an everyday emotion of life leads people to over-normalize it. Often unappreciated is that clinically significant depression constitutes not just a passing state of depression but an enduring constellation of associated symptoms that together render it so burdensome if not painful (American Psychiatric Association 2013). Depressive disorders get lost somewhere between misunderstanding or unawareness on the part of the public and miscommunication and possibly even lack of communication on the part of mental health and public health professionals

Schizophrenia

Schizophrenia represents a lifelong condition characterized by recurrent to chronic psychosis (hallucinations and/or delusions) and underlying and usually entrenched problems with self-care, socializing, and work (American Psychiatric Association 2013). In the 2010 Global Burden of Disease study, schizophrenia was the 4th leading cause of YLD and fifth leading contributor to DALY among all of the mental and substance use disorders (Whiteford et al. 2013). On the other hand, its overall worldwide prevalence over a twelve-month period has been placed around 4 per 1,000 (Saha et al. 2005). This roughly makes schizophrenia one order of magnitude less common than Major Depression.

Yet, experience repeatedly shows how the limited resources that countries devote to mental health care typically get directed towards patients with schizophrenia, even if they are wholly inadequate for the care of such a debilitating condition. It is individuals with schizophrenia and related chronic mental illnesses who are usually the most visible faces of mental health problems in low resource settings around the world (whether or not people know the name or existence of the diagnosis). There are certainly a host of reasons for this, including sufferers' often profound levels of personal and social disorganization and potential for agitation as well as schizophrenia's chronicity. We have repeatedly seen how communities worldwide tend to feel haunted by the presence of schizophrenia, leaving them to cloister those plagued by it, along with much of the public's mental health funding, in remote mental institutions.

Anxiety disorders

Anxiety disorders involve anxiety that has reached a 'clinical' level due to its intensity, frequency, or dysfunctionality. This can encompass problems with worrying too much and about too many things (Generalized Anxiety Disorder), inappropriate panic attacks (Panic Disorder), being too socially anxious (Social Phobia), and obsessions and compulsions (Obsessive Compulsive Disorder). A related problem is the pathologically persistent state of a fear and associated emotions that can occur in response to a traumatic experience known as Post-Traumatic Stress Disorder (PTSD) (American Psychiatric Association 2013).

Anxiety disorders are thought to be common around the world, and accounted for the second most common psychiatric cause of YLD in the 2010 GBD study behind Major Depression (Whiteford et al. 2013). As for regional variations, we are familiar with one study that found overall current worldwide prevalence of all anxiety disorders to be 7.3 percent, while finding the rate in African cultures to be 5.3 percent compared to 10.4 percent in Anglo-European cultures (Baxter et al. 2013). A similar trend is suggested by a 2009 publication of the WHO World Mental Health Survey, where the United States had the highest lifetime (31 percent) and 12-month (19 percent) prevalence of anxiety disorders (Kessler et al. 2009). On the other hand, the 2010 GBD study found that people from conflict ridden regions were 60 percent more likely than those living free of conflict to suffer from an anxiety disorder. In fact, one study of diverse post-conflict settings in Algeria, Cambodia, Gaza, and Ethiopia found rates of PTSD in the range of 15.8–37.4 percent, significantly higher than that of Western community samples (De Jong et al. 2001).

In practice, we have not found that anxiety disorders receive much, if any, clinical attention around the world. There are even criticisms that PTSD in particular is a Western construct that over-medicalizes suffering related to problematic life circumstances around much of the world (Summerfield 2001). Mental health colleagues working in low and middle income countries have expressed to us that they believe clinical anxiety is under-recognized and under-treated. They also voice feeling it themselves in the form of work-related stress that inevitably arises in their dire work circumstances. We have even met people who expressed wonderment that anxiety was something that could be treated, having taken it to be an inalterable fact of human life. Altogether, our impression is that for many people, finding the dividing line between expectable anxieties related to the stresses of life and abnormal anxiety is not easy. Many people do not even consider that such a line could exist.

Substance use disorders

Alcohol and substance use disorders were the third and fourth most common contributors to DALY (behind depressive and anxiety disorders) among the mental and substance use disorders in 2010. Alcohol in particular stands out among all mental health conditions as a major worldwide source of both mortality and morbidity. As of 2004, alcohol use disorders contributed to nearly 4 percent of all deaths and 5 percent of disability adjusted life years worldwide (Whiteford et al. 2013). They are therefore considered one of the largest modifiable risk factors contributing to both health and economic problems (Rehm et al. 2009). On the other hand, it is known that there is great variation in the rates of alcohol use around the world, with abstention seen in regions such as the Middle East and Northern Africa and the most destructive patterns of drinking found in places such as Central and Eastern Europe and portions of Sub-Saharan Africa and South America (Shield et al. 2013).

Illicit drugs are estimated to have contributed to 0.9 percent of worldwide DALY in 2010, making them the 19th leading risk factor for disability adjusted life years. Although marijuana is by far the most commonly used illicit drug in the world, opioids and amphetamine use disorders are most common. Ultimately, opiate dependence was the largest contributor to the global burden associated with illicit drugs (Degenhardt et al. 2013).

In fact, we have yet to work in a low resource setting where alcohol, drugs, or both were not seen as major problems by our medical colleagues and community members alike. Even in places where alcohol is forbidden on religious grounds, such as Iran, use of other drugs such as opioids proliferates (Farhoudian et al. 2013). Psychiatric systems often seem to deal almost as much with substance related disorders as they do schizophrenia, as in the case of Saint Vincent and the Grenadines (World Health Organization and the Ministry of Health of Saint Vincent and the Grenadines 2009). We have found that requests for assistance with addressing a community's alcohol or drugs abound.

Suicide

The WHO estimates that for the year 2020, 1.3 million people will die from suicide and 10–20 times more will attempt suicide. This would translate into 1 death every 20 seconds and 1 attempt every 1–2 seconds (Bertolote & Fleischmann 2002). Moreover, data from 2004 indicates that 84 percent of all suicides in the world take place in low and middle income countries, with India and China alone accounting for 49 percent (Phillips & Cheng 2012). Suicide rates generally correlate with both the prevalence of psychiatric conditions, especially depressive and alcohol use disorders, and the local cultural, social, and economic context (Levi, La Vecchia, & Saraceno 2003). However, the latter may well play a more primary role in such places as China, where studies consistently show that nearly half of suicides occur in individuals without mental illness (Phillips 2010).

Elsewhere as in the Western world, suicide often captures the popular imagination. It, along with the potential for violence towards others, is significantly associated in peoples' minds with mental illness, if not equated with it. Suicide also tends to be among the highest concerns people have about the mentally ill, even if their views of the overall dangerousness and unpredictability of psychiatric patients are extreme (Winer et al. 2013). The scarcity of inpatient psychiatric facilities and of mental health professionals in low and middle income countries then beget circumstances where suicidal individuals are 'helped' by such crude means as locking them to a bedpost or a tree.

Child and adolescent mental disorders

Between 1990 and 2010, the global burden in DALY associated with anorexia increased by 65.7 percent, pervasive developmental disorders increased by 29.5 percent, and disorders such as attention-deficit hyperactivity disorder and conduct disorder increased by 14.1 percent (Murray et al. 2012). Overall, however, country or region specific data on child mental health needs is felt to be nearly non-existent for much of the developing world (Maughan 2013). This is especially the case in sub-Saharan Africa (Okasha 2002). As such, child mental health issues receive even less attention than adult mental health issues in low and middle income countries and other low resource settings (Morris et al. 2011). It is therefore not surprising that one of the top five 'grand challenges in mental health' according to a comprehensive survey of researchers, clinicians, policymakers, and other mental health stakeholders was the improvement of children's access to evidence based mental health care (Collins et al. 2011).

Child mental health services are in even greater demand than those for adults in much of the world. We find that requests for help with child and adolescent mental health care are roughly as common as those for help with substance use problems.

Mental health and tropical diseases

The overlap of mental illness and tropical diseases constitutes an area of concern unique to the developing world. Neglected tropical diseases such as leprosy and lymphatic filariasis are associated with mental health problems, an association attributed to the social impact of these often disabling and disfiguring illnesses. Sufferers experience social stigma and employment discrimination as well as outright human rights violations, the consequences of which can include depressive and other psychiatric conditions (Litt, Baker, & Molyneux 2012).

In regions of the world where falciparum malaria is endemic, cerebral malaria is of particular concern. Fatal in 15–20 percent of cases, cerebral malaria leaves survivors with a range of neurological sequelae, including cognitive problems. Children are especially vulnerable to this outcome and may be left with intellectual, communication, and behavioral problems that get misdiagnosed as problems such as autism or ADHD (Mishra & Newton 2009).

The treatment gap

A discussion about the worldwide burden of mental illness would be incomplete without returning to the issue raised in the Introduction about the extent of this burden which goes unattended. The 'treatment gap' quantifies the difference between the prevalence of a disease and the proportion of affected individuals who receive care. A review of community based mental health surveys from around the world found the following treatment gaps among the various adult disorders: schizophrenia, 32 percent; Major Depression, 56 percent; Dysthymia, 56 percent; Bipolar Disorder (manic-depression), 50 percent; Panic Disorder, 56 percent; Generalized Anxiety Disorder, 58 percent; OCD, 57 percent; and alcohol use disorders, 78 percent (Kohn et al. 2004). As the investigators lacked data about almost all of the conditions in the typically low income regions of Africa, South Asia, and the Eastern Mediterranean, these glaring numbers are probably underestimates. But, for comparison, the treatment gap for American adults with any mental disorder in the United States was 67.1 percent in 2001–2003 (Kessler et al. 2005).

As already discussed, international data on child mental health needs is felt to be virtually non-existent. On the other hand, data from the United States is available and paints a picture of a yawning child mental health treatment gap of 80 percent in children and adolescents aged 6 to 17 years old in need of treatment even in a leading high-income country. Importantly, being Latino or uninsured were risk factors for lacking access to mental health care, reminding us that the US is not immune to issues of mental health access (Kataoka, Zhang, & Wells 2002).

Stigma

Finally, this discussion of epidemiology must be punctuated with consideration about societal stigma towards mental health issues. There are population level studies of mental health stigma or 'attitude research' available. Reviews of these studies across countries suggest that a substantial number of people tend to be unable to identify a psychiatric illness in others; to believe the mentally ill need help; to regard them as dangerous and unpredictable and to therefore distance themselves from them; and to be more rejecting of people with alcohol or drug use problems and schizophrenia as compared to clinical depression or anxiety (Angermeyer & Dietrich 2006). There was also a trend towards non-Westerners being less empathic towards the mentally ill. On the other hand, a study of Canadian community members, schizophrenia researchers, and medical students found them to be well informed and understanding about people with schizophrenia while also noting that as social distance between respondents and the putative schizophrenic was reduced, discomfort and especially fears about their dangerousness escalated (Thompson et al. 2002).

One far ranging study looked at attitudes towards both schizophrenia and major depression in 16 countries as diverse as the US, Iceland, and Bangladesh. They identified five core beliefs that they described as the 'backbone' of stigma, as follows: sufferers may be impulsive, should not care for children, should not teach children, and are self-injurious while respondents endorsed that they would be unwilling to have them as an in-law. These beliefs held for both schizophrenia and depression, even if in the latter case they were less common, and across all countries irrespective of income level (Pescosolido et al. 2013).

There is good reason to believe that the mental health treatment gap derives in no small part from the influence of stigmatized views on all segments of society spanning government leaders, policymakers, health care professionals, and community members. For example, stigma may explain why Sam might not have even contemplated whether he was suffering from a mental health condition. And, although 'stigma' sometimes appears to be proffered too readily and explained too little as the cure-all explanation for the treatment gap, thoughtful discussions and research about it are the pathways to making headway in understanding and addressing it.

Conclusions

The global mental health practitioner can take several points away from the review of the epidemiology of worldwide mental health inspired by Sam. These can be thought of as a checklist of considerations:

✓ Given the breadth of unmet mental health problems worldwide, how prepared are you, the mental health clinician, to step into circumstances where you will be seen as the expert in areas that might otherwise extend beyond your customary area of practice? This could encompass child mental health in particular, addictions, tropical diseases, or even adult psychiatric disorders that one is less conversant in due to their personal practice focus. If you are not comfortable in any particular area, you should make arrangements to coordinate with willing specialists back home, even if by phone, email, or other remote means.

✓ Can a clinician acting as such make the most difference amid so much need? We have found that it is hard for those trained as clinicians to switch gears and resist treating patients. However, if you can do so and are permitted to do so, then teaching and training local professionals and even community members about the principles of basic mental health could leave behind something with an enduring impact at the population level.

✓ Given the prevalence of mental health stigma around the world, could you best maximize your impact on any given community by working in the role of an advocate and educator for mental health (see Chapter 4)? Host communities are invariably accepting of and hospitable towards visiting mental health professionals, but such politeness does not ensure their being accepting and hospitable towards mental health (especially after you leave).

✓ In localities where there is an information vacuum regarding population level mental health needs, as, for example, is inevitably the case regarding the epidemiology of child mental health, are you able and willing to help conduct a needs assessment and research the issue before practicing? Local hosts in the health or mental health professions or the non-governmental sectors will often implore you to focus on certain needs or populations, and you will have to decide whether to deem their request suffices as an assessment, to gauge the authority of their information, or to collect more information.

✓ How prepared are you to work in a multi-disciplinary fashion? As will be discussed later, the absence of abundant mental health resources requires working with non-traditional partners. Here we especially highlight the increasing prevalence and burden of NCD and urge you to collaborate, even co-locate, with medical professionals in addressing NCD and mental health at once. It is far more likely that patients will show up for diabetes or blood pressure checks than for mental health appointments.

✓ Finally, learn about your host country and community before you do anything else in the field, especially teach or otherwise share your psychiatric expertise. Remember the background we provided about Sam at the outset of the chapter and extrapolate it to the level of a country—learn about it as you would a patient. All the epidemiology in the world will fall flat if it is not applied within a local context and culture.

References

American Psychiatric Association 2013, *Diagnostic and Statistical Manual of the American Psychiatric Association*, Arlington, VA, American Psychiatric Association.

Angermeyer, M.C. & Dietrich, S. 2006, 'Public beliefs about and attitudes towards people with mental illness: a review of population studies,' *Acta Psychiatrica Scandinavica*, vol. 113, no. 3, pp. 163–179.

Baxter, A.J., Scott, K.M., Vos, T., & Whiteford, H.A. 2013, 'Global prevalence of anxiety disorders: a systematic review and meta-regression,' *Psychological Medicine*, vol. 43, no. 5, pp. 897–910.

Beaglehole, R., Ebrahim, S., Reddy, S., Voute, J., Leeder, S., & Chronic Disease Action Group 2007, 'Prevention of chronic diseases: a call to action,' *The Lancet*, vol. 370, no. 9605, pp. 2152–2157.

Bertolote, J.M. & Fleischmann, A. 2002, 'A global perspective in the epidemiology of suicide,' *Suicidology*, vol. 7, no. 2, pp. 6–8.

Bromet, E., Andrade, L.H., Hwang, I., Sampson, N.A., Alonso, J., de Girolamo, G., et al. 2011, 'Cross-national epidemiology of DSM-IV major depressive episode,' *BMC Medicine*, vol. 9, no. 1, p. 90.

Collins, P.Y., Patel, V., Joestl, S.S., March, D., Insel, T.R., Daar, A.S., Scientific Advisory Board and the Executive Committee of the Grand Challenges on Global Mental Health, et al. 2011, 'Grand challenges in global mental health,' *Nature*, vol. 475, no. 7354, pp. 27–30.

De Jong, J.T., Komproe, I.H., Van Ommeren, M., El Masri, M., Araya, M., Khaled, N., et al. 2001, 'Lifetime events and posttraumatic stress disorder in 4 postconflict settings,' *JAMA: The Journal of the American Medical Association,* vol. 286, no. 5, pp. 555–562.

Degenhardt, L., Whiteford, H.A., Ferrari, A.J., Baxter, A.J., Charlson, F.J., Hall, W.D., et al. 2013, 'Global burden of disease attributable to illicit drug use and dependence: findings from the Global Burden of Disease Study 2010,' *The Lancet,* vol. 382, no. 9904, pp. 1564–1574.

Farhoudian, A., Hajebi, A., Bahramnejad, A., & Katz, C.L. 2013, 'The perspective of psychosocial support a decade after Bam earthquake: achievements and challenges,' *The Psychiatric Clinics of North America,* vol. 36, no. 3, pp. 385–402.

Ferrari, A.J., Charlson, F.J., Norman, R.E., Patten, S.B., Freedman, G., Murray, C.J., et al. 2013a, 'Burden of depressive disorders by country, sex, age, and year: findings from the Global Burden of Disease Study 2010,' *PLoS Medicine,* vol. 10, no. 11, p. e1001547.

Ferrari, A.J., Somerville, A.J., Baxter, A.J., Norman, R., Patten, S.B., Vos, T., & Whiteford, H.A. 2013b, 'Global variation in the prevalence and incidence of major depressive disorder: a systematic review of the epidemiological literature,' *Psychological Medicine,* vol. 43, no. 3, pp. 471–481.

Kataoka, S.H., Zhang, L., & Wells, K.B. 2002, 'Unmet need for mental health care among US children: variation by ethnicity and insurance status,' *The American Journal of Psychiatry,* vol. 159, no. 9, pp. 1548–1555.

Kessler, R.C., Aguilar-Gaxiola, S., Alonso, J., Chatterji, S., Lee, S., Ormel, J., et al. 2009, 'The global burden of mental disorders: an update from the WHO World Mental Health (WMH) surveys,' *Epidemiologia e Psichiatria Sociale,* vol. 18, no. 1, pp. 23–33.

Kessler, R.C., Demler, O., Frank, R.G., Olfson, M., Pincus, H.A., Walters, E.E., et al. 2005, 'Prevalence and treatment of mental disorders, 1990 to 2003,' *The New England Journal of Medicine,* vol. 352, no. 24, pp. 2515–2523.

Kohn, R., Saxena, S., Levav, I., & Saraceno, B. 2004, 'The treatment gap in mental health care,' *Bulletin of the World Health Organization,* vol. 82, no. 11, pp. 858–866.

Levi, F., La Vecchia, C., & Saraceno, B. 2003, 'Global suicide rates,' *European Journal of Public Health,* vol. 13, no. 2, pp. 97–98.

Litt, E., Baker, M.C., & Molyneux, D. 2012, 'Neglected tropical diseases and mental health: a perspective on comorbidity,' *Trends in Parasitology,* vol. 28, no. 5, pp. 195–201.

Magnusson, R. 2009, 'Rethinking global health challenges: towards a "Global Compact" for reducing the burden of chronic disease,' *Public Health,* vol. 123, no. 3, pp. 265–274.

Maughan, B. 2013, 'Counting the cost: estimating the burden of child mental health,' *Journal of Child Psychology and Psychiatry, and Allied Disciplines,* vol. 54, no. 12, pp. 1261–1262.

Mishra, S.K. & Newton, C.R. 2009, 'Diagnosis and management of the neurological complications of falciparum malaria,' *Nature Reviews Neurology,* vol. 5, no. 4, pp. 189–198.

Morris, J., Belfer, M., Daniels, A., Flisher, A., Ville, L., Lora, A., & Saxena, S. 2011, 'Treated prevalence of and mental health services received by children and adolescents in 42 low- and middle-income countries,' *Journal of Child Psychology and Psychiatry, and Allied Disciplines,* vol. 52, no. 12, pp. 1239–1246.

Murray, C.J., Vos, T., Lozano, R., Naghavi, M., Flaxman, A.D., Michaud, C., et al. 2012, 'Disability-adjusted life years (DALYs) for 291 diseases and injuries in 21 regions, 1990–2010: a systematic analysis for the Global Burden of Disease Study 2010,' *The Lancet,* vol. 380, no. 9859, pp. 2197–2223.

Ngui, E.M., Khasakhala, L., Ndetei, D., & Roberts, L.W. 2010, 'Mental disorders, health inequalities and ethics: a global perspective,' *International Review of Psychiatry,* vol. 22, no. 3, pp. 235–244.

Okasha, A. 2002, 'Mental health in Africa: the role of the WPA,' *World Psychiatry: Official Journal of the World Psychiatric Association (WPA)*, vol. 1, no. 1, pp. 32–35.

Pescosolido, B.A., Medina, T.R., Martin, J.K., & Long, J.S. 2013, 'The "backbone" of stigma: identifying the global core of public prejudice associated with mental illness,' *American Journal of Public Health*, vol. 103, no. 5, pp. 853–860.

Phillips, M.R. 2010, 'Rethinking the role of mental illness in suicide,' *The American Journal of Psychiatry*, vol. 167, no. 7, pp. 731–733.

Phillips, M.R. & Cheng, H.G. 2012, 'The changing global face of suicide,' *The Lancet*, vol. 379, no. 9834, pp. 2318–2319.

Rehm, J., Mathers, C., Popova, S., Thavorncharoensap, M., Teerawattananon, Y., & Patra, J. 2009, 'Global burden of disease and injury and economic cost attributable to alcohol use and alcohol-use disorders,' *The Lancet*, vol. 373, no. 9682, pp. 2223–2233.

Sachs, J.D. & McArthur, J.W. 2005, 'The millennium project: a plan for meeting the Millennium Development Goals,' *The Lancet*, vol. 365, no. 9456, pp. 347–353.

Saha, S., Chant, D., Welham, J., & McGrath, J. 2005, 'A systematic review of the prevalence of schizophrenia,' *PLoS Medicine*, vol. 2, no. 5, p. e141.

Shield, K.D., Rylett, M., Gmel, G., Gmel, G., Kehoe-Chan, T.A., & Rehm, J. 2013, 'Global alcohol exposure estimates by country, territory and region for 2005—a contribution to the Comparative Risk Assessment for the 2010 Global Burden of Disease Study,' *Addiction*, vol. 108, no. 5, pp. 912–922.

Summerfield, D. 2001, 'The invention of post-traumatic stress disorder and the social usefulness of a psychiatric category,' *British Medical Journal (International edn)*, vol. 322, no. 7278, p. 95.

Thompson, A.H., Stuart, H., Bland, R.C., Arboleda-Florez, J., Warner, R., & Dickson, R.A. 2002, 'Attitudes about schizophrenia from the pilot site of the WPA worldwide campaign against the stigma of schizophrenia,' *Social Psychiatry and Psychiatric Epidemiology*, vol. 37, no. 10, pp. 475–482.

United Nations 2014, *Millenium Development Goals and Beyond 2015: Background*. Available: www.un.org/millenniumgoals/bkgd.shtml (accessed January 20, 2014).

Whiteford, H.A., Degenhardt, L., Rehm, J., Baxter, A.J., Ferrari, A.J., Erskine, H.E., et al. 2013, 'Global burden of disease attributable to mental and substance use disorders: findings from the Global Burden of Disease Study 2010,' *The Lancet*, vol. 382, no. 9904, pp. 1575–1586.

Winer, R.A., Morris-Patterson, A., Smart, Y., Bijan, I., & Katz, C.L. 2013, 'Knowledge of and attitudes toward mental illness among primary care providers in Saint Vincent and the Grenadines,' *The Psychiatric Quarterly*, vol. 84, no. 3, pp. 395–406.

World Health Organization 2014a, *Malaria*. Available: www.who.int/gho/malaria/en/index.html (accessed January 20, 2014).

World Health Organization 2014b, *Tuberculosis*. Available: www.who.int/gho/tb/en/index.html (accessed January 20, 2014).

World Health Organization 2014c, *Neglected Tropical Diseases*. Available: www.who.int/gho/neglected_diseases/en/index.html (accessed January 20, 2014).

World Health Organization and the Ministry of Health of Saint Vincent and the Grenadines 2009, *WHO AIMS Report on the Mental Health System of Saint Vincent and the Grenadines*, World Health Organization, Geneva.

Chapter 2

Human resources

Sam arrived at the hospital hoping to learn what was causing his fatigue. After waiting for five hours, it was finally Sam's turn to see the doctor. It had been months since he last slept well or was able to say that he felt anything but exhaustion when waking up. The doctor approached him apologetically, informing him that he could not check Sam's blood sugar, as their machine was currently out of order. It would be weeks or maybe months before they could get it repaired. However, the good news: his blood smear showed no signs of malarial infection. He urged Sam to not worry so much; it was probably nothing that some rest and a good diet wouldn't improve. This was reassuring, for now. As Sam walked home through the dusty streets filled with motorcycles, people, and stray dogs, his brief feeling of hope gradually soured. How had he forgotten to tell his doctor that these days he could miss breakfast, lunch, and even dinner without feeling hungry? He would love to follow his doctor's advice if he only knew how.

It is an all too common scenario that we have imagined, where patients are incorrectly diagnosed or where psychiatric problems are easily overlooked. Sam seems to know that something is amiss but lacks the ability to make the connection between his emotional state and his physical condition. Unfortunately, his doctor seems to lack that very same ability, rendering him an inadequate diagnostician. Technological advances have revolutionized the field of diagnostic and interventional medicine over the last 100 years (Porter 1999), but during that same timeframe psychiatrists have hardly changed their diagnostic approach. A patient is still assessed using, for the most part, the basic tools that we all possess: our senses, intellect, and ability to communicate. While the development of psychotropic medication has lead to significant advances in the treatment of mental illness, the very qualities we use to assess a patient are also the ones we often employ to help them. At this point in time, psychotherapy can only take place between human beings. Without the availability of human beings to utilize their diagnostic and therapeutic tools, mental health cannot be addressed.

In this chapter we will explore the importance of human resources in the treatment of the psychiatric illness, along with the vast shortages all too common in the developing world. Following a description of the current state of psychiatric human resources, we will discuss ideas on how access to mental health care can be strengthened by introducing the concept of task shifting. Finally, we invite the reader to contemplate a common scenario and think about how effective collaboration can improve access to psychiatric human resources.

Who is providing mental health care?

In a paper by Kakuma et al., which uses The World Health Report 2006 as a springboard, the mental health care workforce is described as including three distinct groups of individuals. The first is comprised of highly trained specialist workers such as psychiatrists, neurologists, mental health nurses, psychologists, mental health social workers, and occupational therapists. These professionals all have some form of psychiatric training in common and, with the exception of nurses, are a rarity in low resource settings. The second group includes health workers without specific psychiatric training, such as doctors (of varying specialties), nurses and lay health workers, affected individuals, and caregivers. The last group consists of other professionals without health training, such as teachers and community-level workers (Kakuma et al. 2011; World Health Organization 2006b).

The availability of human resources in the mental health sector correlates directly with any given country's income level. Low income countries only have an average of 1.3 mental health human resources per 100,000 population, whereas high income countries have an average of 50.8 mental health workers per 100,000 population (World Health Organization 2011). Bearing in mind that there have been few changes in the availability of human resources in low income countries between 2005 and 2011 (Kakuma et al. 2011), in a country like Nepal in 2006, with an estimated population of 27 million, this statistic would translate to roughly 360 mental health care workers. However, in reality there were a mere 147 mental health care workers in Nepal in 2006, less than half of the world average (World Health Organization 2006a).

Nurses

Overall, nurses represent the largest group of mental health professionals worldwide. In low income countries there is an average of 1 psychiatric nurse for 240,000 people. In lower-middle income countries that number improves to roughly 1 nurse per 35,000 people, but remains vastly insufficient overall (World Health Organization 2011) (see Figure 2.1).

In a study including 58 low and middle income countries, a shortage of 127,575 mental health nurses was identified (Bruckner et al. 2011). Mental health nurses play a valuable role in the implementation of mental health care as their contributions become increasingly varied and complex. In addition to direct patient care, nurses also have administrative and policy-making responsibilities. According to the WHO *Nurses in Mental Health Atlas* 2007, which compiled survey data from international mental health nurses, they may even take on the roles of physicians and psychiatrists in low resource settings, prescribing medications, running inpatient wards and conducting outpatient care (World Health Organization 2007). They are the most frequently encountered health care workers in low resource settings and are therefore often called on to work in areas outside of their expertise. The latter two issues can create a sense of frustration as they are often asked to make decisions

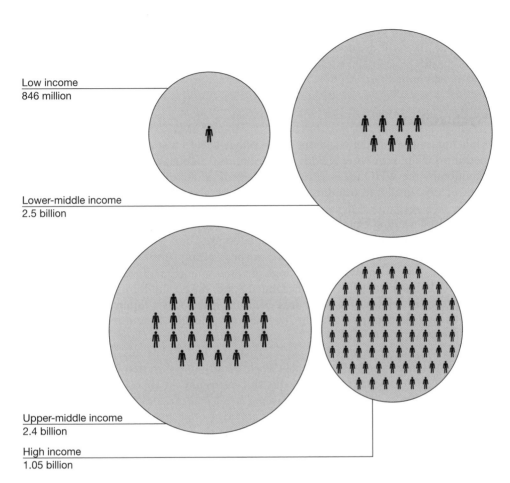

Low income
846 million

Lower-middle income
2.5 billion

Upper-middle income
2.4 billion

High income
1.05 billion

Figure 2.1 Mental health nurse density by population and income-level countries

👤 = 0.42 mental health nurses/100,000 population
Source: World Health Organization 2011; World Bank 2014

without being given proper authority to do so. In many cases though nurses are given direct authority to prescribe or continue medications, making them invaluable to the delivery of psychiatric care in the absence of physicians. In several of our collaborative sites, we have witnessed nurses providing the foundation of psychiatric care. They have played the part of psychiatrists running a comprehensive outpatient and community outreach program, consultants in a hospital devoid of any psychiatric care, de facto substance abuse counselors, as well as hospital administrators.

With nurses being such a versatile and precious human resource, how do we explain their prodigious scarcity? As is the case with all human resources in the mental health field, the lack of prioritization in health care budgets significantly impacts the availability of professionals. Furthermore, the lack of financial or other incentives prevents nurses from receiving specialized training. These factors, combined with stigma and lack of basic psychiatric training, render psychiatry an undesirable subspecialty (World Health Organization 2007). Improved awareness of psychiatric illness, along with systematic de-stigmatization during their training, could alleviate this notion. We will discuss at the end of the chapter more in detail how the global mental health practitioner could play a role in promoting the employment of nurses, directly and indirectly.

Psychiatrists

While nurses provide the backbone for psychiatric care worldwide, psychiatrists are needed to help supervise, guide, and train the mental health workforce. Their definition by the WHO reads as follows: 'A medical doctor who has had at least two years of post-graduate training in psychiatry at a recognized teaching institution leading to a recognized degree or diploma' (World Health Organization 2011). A high level of training enables them to provide comprehensive care while hopefully being able to multi-task as administrators, advocates, and policymakers.

As expected though, psychiatrists are in short supply, not only in the developing world, but also in many areas of high income countries (Health Resources and Services Administration 2014). In the United States the Health Resources and Services Administration defines a shortage area as a region that has a ration equal or greater than 1 psychiatrist per 30,000 population (Health Resources and Services Administration 2014). The WHO numbers in high income countries support this scale, showing an average of 8.59 psychiatrists per 100,000 people, or the equivalent of 2.6 psychiatrists per 30,000 people (World Health Organization 2011). Keeping in mind epidemiologic data for the US, this still seems like an abhorrently low number. If the 12-month prevalence of schizophrenia is 1.1 percent, and of bipolar disorder is 2.6 percent, along with the 12-month prevalence of major depressive disorder (6.7 percent) and panic disorder (2.7 percent), then of those 30,000 people, we would expect at least 4,000 to have an impairing psychiatric illness (Kessler et al. 2005). This figure of course does not capture a host of other disorders that lead to psychiatric morbidity (substance abuse disorders, dementia, etc.). So, in a high income country, with an average of 2.6 psychiatrists per 30,000 people, an average psychiatrist would have a caseload of 1,500 patients. In order for the psychiatrist working a 50-hour week to see each patient on an outpatient monthly basis, he or she would have to see one patient every 7.5 minutes. In contrast, a study by Olfson et al. (1999) showed that the mean psychiatric visit duration in the US in 1995 was found to be 38.1 minutes.

Now, let us look at the data for low resource settings. Low income countries are estimated to have an average of 0.05 psychiatrists per 100,000 population or the equivalent of 1 psychiatrist for 2 million people (World Health Organization 2011). Using the scenario above and worldwide point prevalence of only two psychiatric disorders, major depressive disorder (4.7 percent) and schizophrenia (0.4 percent) (Ferrari et al. 2013; Saha et al. 2005), we arrive at minimum of 5,100 patients per 100,000 people. Given that there is only an average of 1 psychiatrist per 2 million people in low income countries, the psychiatrist would be faced by a minimum caseload of 102,000 people. These numbers help us come to a clearer understanding of why mental health nurses are required to play the role of psychiatrists in these low resource settings.

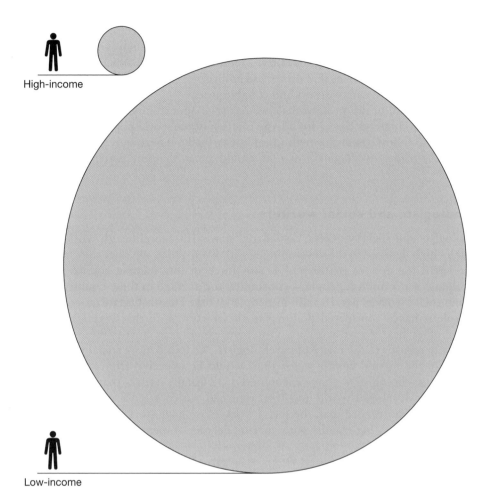

High-income

Low-income

Figure 2.2 Estimates for current psychiatrist-to-patient ratio in high- and low-income
countries. High-income countries have 1 psychiatrist for ~12,000 people while
low-income countries have 1 psychiatrist for 2 million people.

Similarly to mental health nurses, psychiatrists are not well funded in low income
settings. The trivial proportion of health care budgets being allotted to mental health
(World Health Organization 2011), along with the relatively high cost of physicians
(compared to nurses and other health care workers), creates few opportunities and
financial incentives for psychiatrists to seek work in these countries. Few graduates
from low income countries practice in their home country, as conditions and salaries
in higher-income areas are much more desirable (Gureje et al. 2009). This 'brain-
drain' phenomenon is common among all types of professionals in health care, and
also outside of the health care industry.

We have collaborated with psychiatrists who have remained in or returned to their
country after receiving training elsewhere. We were universally impressed by their
ambition and commitment and have witnessed what it means to be the only psychiatrist

in an entire country. In fact, the term 'the only psychiatrist in the country' is something we have encountered too many times, and in scales that are difficult to imagine. The sheer magnitude of care that needs to be provided can be and definitely is overwhelming at times. And it is not surprising that there are few, if any, professionals lining up to take these positions. The ones that do remain and persist can only do so with the help of other mental health care workers and collaborators.

As global mental health professionals we have the opportunity to come to the aid of these few psychiatrists caring for a large fraction of the world population. Further discussion will follow about the methods of bolstering human resources, but for now we invite the reader to imagine how they would assist 'the only psychiatrist in the country.'

Psychologists and social workers

Psychologists and social workers, considered specialist mental health workers, are in equally high demand in the developing world. Even added together they make up only a small fraction of the mental health force in low income countries. One psychologist per 5 million people is considered the average in these countries as is only one social worker per 10 million people (World Health Organization 2011). Their role is hence considered minimal in these settings, further highlighting the need for other health care workers. Our own experiences mirror these findings, especially in regards to the rarity of psychologists. We found more social workers to be active in the mental health sector than would be expected from the statistics above. The psychologists we have encountered are usually natives that have trained abroad in the developed world and then returned out of a sense of duty to their home country. Contrary to that, the social workers we have worked with tend to be more locally trained, but usually with varying degrees of mental health skills.

Non-psychiatrist physicians

There are an estimated 0.06 non-psychiatrist physicians per 100,000 population providing mental health care in low income countries (World Health Organization 2011). This figure is slightly higher than the amount of psychiatrists practicing in these settings (0.05/100,000), so we can therefore assume that psychiatric patients have more access to these physicians. As the amount of psychiatrists increases according to country income level, so do the non-specialists, but at a lower rate (see Table 2.1).

Table 2.1 Comparison of psychiatrists and non-psychiatrists providing mental health care by country income levels per 100,000 population

Income level	Psychiatrists	Non-psychiatrist physicians
Low	0.05	0.06
Lower-middle	0.54	0.21
Upper-middle	2.03	0.87
High	8.59	1.49

We have come across these physicians in our own global health work and have noticed that they tend to be non-psychiatrists who show an interest in the psychiatric population, or were available to provide care when no one else was. We observed them to be extremely dedicated but also highly aware of their lack of psychiatric training. In all cases, they seemed eager to expand their knowledge and collaborate with us.

In low income and middle income countries, as suggested by evidence, one of the best ways to enhance psychiatric care is to provide support for primary care professionals (Desjarlais 1996; World Health Organization 2001). These physicians are an important resource for providing initial contact with psychiatric patients. They are known and trusted in the community and can be instrumental in guiding patients towards proper care (Patel et al. 2008). Enlisting their support can be achieved by helping them identify and treat psychiatric patients through training and assistance by available mental health providers. As we saw in the vignette above, Sam's doctor unfortunately did not add depression to the list of differential diagnoses and missed an opportunity to help his patient. This is all too common given that less than a third of clinically significant morbidity is detected in primary care, and that mental health training comprises only an average of 2 percent of physicians' undergraduate training hours worldwide (Ciston & Von Korff 1995; World Health Organization 2006a).

Community health workers/lay mental health workers

As we will discuss below and in Chapter 6 on psychotherapy, task shifting is an important concept that can help redistribute the available human resources within a workforce. A key component to successful psychiatric care in low resource settings has been the training of lay people and non-psychiatric community health workers in mental health. While the availability of trained mental health staff tends to be low in the developing world there is no shortage whatsoever of lay people. Many programs have shown that lay people can be effectively trained to provide various non-prescriber interventions such as counseling and case management (Bolton et al. 2003; Rahman et al. 2008; Patel et al. 2010). See Chapter 6 for further details regarding the use of lay mental health workers in providing counseling and psychotherapy.

Task shifting

Task shifting can be described as a meaningful redistribution of tasks within a workforce. In the case of global health, this means assigning tasks traditionally fulfilled by higher-trained health care professionals to less highly trained individuals. Taking into consideration the workforce teams as described above, we can see how task shifting is a necessity for providing even a minimum of adequate care to psychiatric patients worldwide. Whether implemented in an organized fashion or not, it is the reason why many of the patients in low resource countries receive any psychiatric care at all.

Examining a psychiatrist's skills and tasks, we can consider the following list:

- Assessment/evaluation: this includes screening
- Diagnosis: more thorough assessment to arrive at a diagnosis

- Initiation of psychotropic medication
- Continuation of psychotropic medication
- Management of psychotropic medication including titration, tapering, discontinuation, and management of side effects
- Management of minor medical comorbidities
- Psychotherapy/counseling, individual and group
- Administration of electroconvulsive treatment (ECT)
- Liaison with other medical professionals
- Supervision
- Research
- Advocacy
- Administration
- Policy development.

Now let us consider which of these tasks and skills can be performed, to a reasonable degree, by non-psychiatrists. Table 2.2 breaks down the categories by level of training needed to perform the tasks. In this scenario, we envision that non-mental health staff have received a reasonable degree of mental health training.

Table 2.2 reveals a considerable amount of work that can be performed by non-specialist staff. If done correctly, one psychiatrist can make a considerable impact by training other staff members to perform some of his or her duties. Providing regular supervision can subsequently ensure a high level of competency and care.

The success of task shifting initiatives depends on various factors, as described by Padmanathan and De Silva (2013). First, efforts should be made to understand whether your target population would accept the help of the workforce. In other words, training lay mental health workers who will not be accepted by the patients (for instance due to lack of confidence in their skills) may prove problematic. Next,

Table 2.2 Psychiatric tasks by level of training

Task	Psychiatrist	Non-psychiatric physician	Mental health nurse	Nurse	Lay mental health worker
Evaluation	+	+	+	+	+
Diagnosis	+	+	+	+/−	
Medication Management	+	+	+/−		
Medical management	+	+			
Counseling	+	+	+	+	+
ECT	+				
Liaison	+	+	+		
Supervision	+		+		
Research	+				
Advocacy	+	+	+		
Administration	+	+	+	+	+
Policy development	+		+		

ensure that managers and other health professionals are willing to cooperate with task-shifting health care workers. Assist the workforce in dealing with the stressors of their new positions as mental health workers and ensure adequate training. Finally, as with any workforce, ensure adequate incentives for health workers to participate. If financial resources are not available, consider career progression or the issuing of certificates and awards as desirable incentives.

Practical implications

The global mental health practitioner seeking to establish a site of care in a developing country should first take stock of the available human resources. The WHO Assessment Instrument for Mental Health Systems (WHO-AIMS) project was designed to capture countries' existing mental health structures and practices. The primary sources for the data were the Ministries of Health in each country or other institutions nominated by them. However, there is no substitute for doing an assessment of the local human resources on the ground. Speaking with health care providers, community leaders, ministers, politicians, and consumers will be the most effective way of determining what resources you can draw from. A strong willingness to collaborate is an essential ingredient in enhancing a mental health program.

The following checklist should serve as a guide to help determine the best use of the available human resources by the global mental health professional.

- ✓ Educate yourself on the availability of human resources via literature, such as WHO-AIMS.
- ✓ Perform on-the-ground evaluation of available resources by speaking and meeting with local stakeholders, health care professionals, and consumers.
- ✓ Remember to include informal resources such as faith healers, religious figures, teachers, organizations, etc. in your assessment.
- ✓ Evaluate whether local resources are being used effectively.
- ✓ Collaborate with existing health care structures to determine best use of the available resources.
- ✓ Consider integrating mental health care into primary care.
- ✓ Consider task shifting as a cost-effective way to improve care.
- ✓ If considering task shifting, determine the acceptability of this intervention within the community.
- ✓ Help empower staff by advocating for their training and employment as psychiatric professionals.

Let us now imagine a different scenario for Sam; one where his care takes a different route because of an effective mental health care model that has been put into place with the help of a global mental health practitioner. Let us assume that the hospital outpatient clinic where Sam is seeing a doctor employs low cost lay health workers who, among other tasks, screen all patients for depression using a simple tool such as the Patient Health Questionnaire (PHQ-9). While Sam was waiting for his doctor, the lay worker asked him questions and registered that Sam scored quite highly. The score was subsequently passed on to Sam's doctor who referred Sam to the regional mental health nurse. While this scenario does not ensure Sam's improvement, his chances of receiving more appropriate care have dramatically increased. Through thoughtful interventions, often at a low cost, providers can grant access to care that can potentially change people's lives for the better. A careful examination of a country's human resources should be the first stop in creating such a change.

References

Bolton, P., Bass, J., Neugebauer, R., Verdeli, H., Clougherty, K.F., Wickramaratne, P., et al. 2003, 'Group interpersonal psychotherapy for depression in rural Uganda: a randomized controlled trial,' *JAMA: The Journal of the American Medical Association*, vol. 289, no. 23, pp. 3117–3124.

Bruckner, T.A., Scheffler, R.M., Shen, G., Yoon, J., Chisholm, D., Morris, J., et al. 2011, 'The mental health workforce gap in low- and middle-income countries: a needs-based approach,' *Bulletin of the World Health Organization*, vol. 89, no. 3, pp. 184–194.

Ciston, T. & Von Korff, M. 1995, 'Primary mental health services: access and provision of care,' in T.B. Üstün & N. Sartorius, 1995, *Mental Illness in General Health Care: An International Study*, John Wiley & Sons, West Sussex, England, p. 347.

Desjarlais, R. 1996, *World Mental Health: Problems and Priorities in Low-income Countries*, Oxford University Press, New York.

Ferrari, A.J., Somerville, A.J., Baxter, A.J., Norman, R., Patten, S.B., Vos, T., & Whiteford, H.A. 2013, 'Global variation in the prevalence and incidence of major depressive disorder: a systematic review of the epidemiological literature,' *Psychological Medicine*, vol. 43, no. 3, pp. 471–481.

Gureje, O., Hollins, S., Botbol, M., Javed, A., Jorge, M., Okech, V., et al. 2009, 'Report of the WPA task force on brain drain,' *World Psychiatry*, vol. 8, no. 2, pp. 115–118.

Health Resources and Services Administration 2014, *Medically Underserved Areas/Populations*. Available: www.hrsa.gov/shortage/mua/index.html (accessed January 23, 2014).

Kakuma, R., Minas, H., van Ginneken, N., Dal Poz, M.R., Desiraju, K., Morris, J.E., et al. 2011, 'Human resources for mental health care: current situation and strategies for action,' *The Lancet*, vol. 378, no. 9803, pp. 1654–1663.

Kessler, R.C., Chiu, W.T., Demler, O., & Walters, E.E. 2005, 'Prevalence, severity, and comorbidity of 12-month DSM-IV disorders in the National Comorbidity Survey Replication,' *Archives of General Psychiatry*, vol. 62, no. 6, p. 617.

Olfson, M., Marcus, S.C., & Pincus, H.A. 1999, 'Trends in office-based psychiatric practice,' *American Journal of Psychiatry*, vol. 156, no. 3, pp. 451–457.

Padmanathan, P. & De Silva, M.J. 2013, 'The acceptability and feasibility of task-sharing for mental healthcare in low and middle income countries: a systematic review,' *Social Science & Medicine*, vol. 97, pp. 82–86.

Patel, V.H., Kirkwood, B.R., Pednekar, S., Araya, R., King, M., Chisholm, D., et al. 2008, 'Improving the outcomes of primary care attenders with common mental disorders in developing countries: a cluster randomized controlled trial of a collaborative stepped care intervention in Goa, India,' *Trials*, vol. 9, no. 4, doi: 10.1186/1745-6215-9-4.

Patel, V., Weiss, H.A., Chowdhary, N., Naik, S., Pednekar, S., Chatterjee, S., et al. 2010, 'Effectiveness of an intervention led by lay health counsellors for depressive and anxiety disorders in primary care in Goa, India (MANAS): a cluster randomised controlled trial,' *The Lancet*, vol. 376, no. 9758, pp. 2086–2095.

Porter, R. 1999, *The Greatest Benefit to Mankind: A Medical History of Humanity*, 1st edn, W.W. Norton & Company, New York.

Rahman, A., Malik, A., Sikander, S., Roberts, C., & Creed, F. 2008, 'Cognitive behaviour therapy-based intervention by community health workers for mothers with depression and their infants in rural Pakistan: a cluster-randomised controlled trial,' *The Lancet,* vol. 372, no. 9642, pp. 902–909.

Saha, S., Chant, D., Welham, J., & McGrath, J. 2005, 'A systematic review of the prevalence of schizophrenia,' *PLoS Medicine,* vol. 2, no. 5, p. e141.

World Bank 2014, *Data | The World Bank*. Available: http://data.worldbank.org/ (accessed January 23, 2014).

World Health Organization 2001, *The World Health Report: 2001: Mental Health: New Understanding, New Hope*, World Health Organization, Geneva.

World Health Organization 2006a, *WHO–AIMS Report on Mental Health System in Nepal*, World Health Organization & Ministry of Health and Population, Nepal. Available: www. who.int/mental_health/evidence/nepal_who_aims_report.pdf (accessed November 1, 2007).

World Health Organization 2006b, *Working Together for Health: The World Health Report 2006*, World Health Organization, Geneva, pp. 3–15.

World Health Organization 2007, *Atlas: Nurses in Mental Health 2007*, World Health Organization, Geneva.

World Health Organization 2011, *Mental Health Atlas 2011*, World Health Organization, Geneva.

Chapter 3

Non-human resources

The photo also captures George, a young pharmacist who works at the same local hospital where Sam was headed. George's responsibilities in the pharmacy include dispensing medication, taking inventory, and ensuring an adequate stock of medications. His pharmacy supplies a few community clinics on the outskirts of the capital as well as the only mental health hospital in the country, located many miles from the town's center. Having grown up during the previous dictatorship and even having spent time in a refugee camp with his parents, George feels very fortunate to have a steady job and income. He remembers all too well how the family struggled while his father was away, his mother having to rely on family members and the community to ensure adequate nutrition for him and his siblings. Helping others in need now seems to be the right thing to do; it is what gives him purpose and integrity. And so George sees his position at the pharmacy as fundamental in being able to give back to the community, to ensure that they receive the medications and treatment they require.

Three doors down the hallway from Sam's doctor, George was busy taking inventory of the pharmacy medications. He had walked to work at a faster pace than usual that day in order to receive an early shipment of the antidepressant amitriptyline, which had been in short supply for the last five weeks. He had found himself calling private pharmacies in the hope they would sell him a few boxes. Despite his efforts, the shortages persisted and were most felt at the mental hospital outside of town. A set of ramshackle buildings partially destroyed during the civil war represent the only psychiatric hospital in the country. It is here that we find our psychiatric patients. Not in the photograph. They are admitted to the hospital for a variety of reasons, but are invariably locked away from sight.

Medications

Medication availability is a key component to the successful implementation of mental health care, and often proves to be a significant barrier in the global health setting. The World Health Organization (WHO) has been publishing a Model List of Essential Medicines (MLEM) since 1977 (WHO 1977). This list was intended to promote the idea that certain medicines are more important than others in order to ensure that resources flow towards populations in need (Laing et al. 2003). The WHO currently defines essential medicines as 'those that satisfy the priority health care needs of the population' and are selected 'with due regard to disease prevalence, evidence on efficacy and safety, and comparative cost-effectiveness' (WHO 2014).

There have been numerous revisions of the publication, which is updated every two years (as of 2014, 18 editions have been published) and hopes to guide countries to adopt this list as part of their own national MLEM. As of 2014 (18th edition), there are 12 core list psychotropic medications in six categories (medicines used for psychotic disorders, depressive disorders, bipolar disorders, anxiety disorders, obsessive compulsive disorders, substance abuse disorders). While it may appear that 12 medications to treat the breadth of mental illness is rather limited, it is imperative to appreciate and understand their versatility in the treatment of several conditions outside of their respective categories. The professionals practicing global mental health should familiarize themselves as much as possible with the applications of these medications. He or she will find that, much like a Swiss Army knife, they can find use in various settings.

Antipsychotic medications (also commonly referred to as *neuroleptics*) are widely used to treat psychotic illnesses such as schizophrenia and schizoaffective disorder, but also have shown to be efficacious in the use of mood disorders such as bipolar disorder and depression. Furthermore, they are also often successfully used to treat delirium, agitation, and other behavioral disturbances (Schatzberg, Cole, & DeBattista 2010). The list includes three older medications (*conventional antipsychotics*: chlorpromazine, fluphenazine, and haloperidol) and one newer medication (*atypical antipsychotic*), which was only recently added to the MLEM: risperidone.

We find two medications in the category of antidepressants: amitriptyline and fluoxetine (well known as the brand name drug *Prozac*). Both medications are efficacious for use in depression but have also been shown to have positive effects on anxiety, when used consistently over several weeks. In addition, amitriptyline can be used to treat various pain conditions, such as migraines and fibromyalgia, as well as bed-wetting in children (nocturnal enuresis) (Schatzberg et al. 2010).

The WHO LEM also includes three medications used for bipolar disorders, more specifically, to prevent mania: carbamazepine, lithium, and valproic acid (WHO 2014). In addition to this use, carbamazepine and valproic acid are highly effective at treating epilepsy and can be used to prevent impulsive aggression and other impulsive behaviors (Schatzberg et al. 2010). Lithium has also been shown to help treat depression when combined with antidepressant medication (Bauer et al. 2010).

The only medication listed in the category of medicines used to treat anxiety is diazepam (well known as the brand name drug *Valium*). For many people, it works to reduce anxiety in a matter of minutes to hours. When used at higher doses, it can also help reduce agitation as well as catatonia and be used to treat insomnia. Furthermore, diazepam is also a highly effective antiepileptic medication and can be life-saving when administered to someone who is having continuous seizures (Schatzberg et al. 2010).

Generally considered to be an anxiety disorder, obsessive compulsive disorder (OCD) is listed as its own category and includes the medication clomipramine. It is also effectively used for depression, but keep in mind that fluoxetine can also be useful to treat OCD (Schatzberg et al. 2010).

Finally, the WHO lists nicotine replacement therapy as the only core medication to treat substance abuse disorders. Methadone, a highly effective and widely used medication to treat opioid addiction, is listed as a complementary medicine as it is usually administered in the setting of a substance abuse program. Interestingly, we have in our own travels never encountered methadone as being part of a national formulary or on pharmacy shelves. There seems to be a dearth of research in this area as literature searches yield barely any articles related to methadone maintenance use in developing countries. This is surprising, given that opioid dependence is the largest contributor among the global burden associated with illicit drugs (Degenhardt et al. 2013).

ECT

While medications play an integral role in the care of the mentally ill, there are other modalities of treatment that can be not only highly effective, but also highly cost-effective. Electroconvulsive therapy (ECT) has been used to treat psychiatric conditions since the 1930s and, after its use briefly declined in the 1960s and 1970s due to the development of psychotropic medication, is now being widely used in over one million patients per year on all continents (Prudic, Olfson, & Sackeim 2001). ECT is a treatment that involves applying an electric current to a patient's head in order to induce a seizure. Other historical procedures that include induction of seizures were effective as well though we now know that it is not only the induction of seizure activity that is considered to be therapeutic. Common psychiatric conditions that are treated with ECT include depression, schizophrenia, and catatonic states (Hales, Yudofsky, & Weiss Roberts 2014). ECT is currently used mostly for the treatment of depression in the United States, Europe, Australia, and New Zealand. Most Asian and African countries, with some exceptions, however tend to utilize the treatment more in patients with schizophrenia (Leiknes, Schweder, & Høie 2012). Although there remains some controversy as to the efficacy of ECT in schizophrenia, it is generally considered effective, safe, and well tolerated. In fact, it is considered one of the only treatments that are safe in vulnerable populations such as the elderly, the medically compromised, and pregnant patients (van Schaik et al. 2012; Lakshmana et al. 2014).

Several variations on electroconvulsive treatment exist, each carrying their own risks and benefits. Original treatments, or *unmodified ECT* as it is now referred to, were administered to fully conscious patients using electrodes placed on both temples. In this form of treatment patients received a brief electric shock resulting in a full-scale convulsion, visible to the clinician or observer. Given the often-severe muscle contractions, this type of procedure can lead to fractures or dislocations. The addition of the muscle relaxant medication succinylcholine, which paralyzes the body during the seizure, led to a much safer outcome. Modern ECT treatments now include the use of a short-acting anesthetic such as methohexital, thiopental, propofol, etomidate, or ketamine to render the patient unconscious during the procedure (Hales et al. 2014).

While modern ECT is considered well tolerated and safe, many countries, including developed and developing, still employ unmodified ECT. Lack of appropriate medications and anesthesia services have been suggested as possible reasons for this (Chanpattana et al. 2010). A large survey of Asian countries showed that 14 out of 23 countries (61 percent) administered unmodified ECT (Chanpattana et al. 2010) while in Japan, generally considered an affluent and highly modernized country, unmodified ECT was utilized in 57 percent of treatments (Chanpattana et al. 2005). Europe generally utilizes modified ECT while in Russia >80 percent of treatments were reported as unmodified (Nelson 2005). The global mental health worker should be prepared to encounter ECT practices that appear sub-optimal and even disturbing. What further intensifies this feeling are the human rights infractions that can occur when ECT is administered without informed consent or even over a patient's objection.

Medications and ECT can play an integral role in the delivery of mental health care. However, without a larger system in place, these treatments cannot be implemented.

Mental health care services

Psychiatric care can be delivered in a variety of settings ranging from the solitary psychiatric hospital far flung from the community to a rural health clinic to a large multi-staged system that spans inpatient, outpatient, and community outreach care. We have encountered each of these settings in our global health work.

When entering a new community, a global mental health practitioner's priority will be to assess the community's existing mental health care services. The question framing further exploration could read as follows:

What are the systems in place to diagnose, treat, or refer psychiatric patients?

The ensuing questions will help guide the assessment in order to provide a comprehensive understanding of a community's access to mental health care:

1   Are patients admitted to a dedicated psychiatric facility?
2   To what extent are services outpatient-based?
3   Is community outreach being done?
4   What are the local mental health laws and policies governing the practices?
5   Is there an infrastructure in place to enable the use of telepsychiatry?

In order to better understand what the global mental health practitioner will encounter, it is helpful to take a look at the World Health Organization Assessment Instrument for Mental Health Systems (WHO-AIMS) reports. The WHO developed an assessment tool to summarize and monitor descriptive data on mental health systems. In one report, 42 low and middle income countries were assessed and their mental health systems analyzed in order to develop plans for strengthening community care and scaling up care for people with mental illness (WHO 2009). While not surprising, the results have uncovered a vast dearth of mental health care in developing countries. The following should provide some background on the questions above:

1   Inpatient care

    a   Community-based inpatient care. Community-based inpatient care refers to the management of acutely ill patients in units that are part of a community-based hospital. They are different from mental hospitals, which are usually freestanding hospitals entirely dedicated to psychiatric care. Low income countries (LICs), such as Haiti and Bangladesh, have an average of 0.37 psychiatric beds per 100,000 people within these community-based hospitals. This number triples for lower-middle income countries (LMICs), such as Belize, Pakistan, and the Philippines to 1.16 beds/100,000 population. Upper-middle income countries (UMICs), such as Mexico, Libya, and China, have an average of 8.95 beds for 100,000 people, roughly 24 times higher than LICs (WHO 2009).

The global mental health worker will therefore most likely encounter few, if any, community-based psychiatric beds. We have found this to be the case in several of our collaborative sites. One such site in a LMIC in Central America had a total of two dedicated psychiatric beds in a room on a general medical floor in the largest community hospital. While the patients there were seen and treated by consulting mental health staff, the setting was otherwise hardly any different from general medical care.

b Mental hospitals. As mentioned, mental hospitals are standalone facilities dedicated to the treatment of the acutely and chronically mentally ill. They have few ties to community-based services, and often provide their own outpatient care/clinics. Similarly to the community-based inpatient care setting, the number of beds per population rises proportionally to income-level. LICs have 0.86 beds per 100,000 population while UMICs have 20 times that amount (18.02 beds/100,000 population). Interestingly, while the number of beds in LICs has risen, UMICs seem to be reducing the number of beds (WHO 2009). The latter is consistent with an overall global trend of shifting psychiatric care away from costly inpatient hospitalization and towards community-based outpatient care. We have personally witnessed this type of deinstitutionalization at our collaborative site in Belize, where the country's only mental hospital, Rockview Hospital, closed down in 2008 in an effort to decentralize psychiatric care and reintegrate the patients back into their respective communities. This step is considered an innovation and modernization as psychiatric care has historically been based around mental hospitals or asylums. When colonial forces established themselves abroad, they brought with them the centralization of psychiatric care. Unfortunately this has often led to dehumanizing and brutal treatment of the mentally ill in institutions where they were quite literally 'locked away' (Porter 1999). However, a shift away from mental institutions can and should only be achieved if proper outpatient care is available (Patel et al. 2014). In Liberia, a low income country of about 3.7 million people, we found one psychiatric hospital with a capacity of 80 beds, located close to the capital of Monrovia, serves as the only inpatient facility in the country. While the conditions in the hospital are less-than-optimal, closing the facility would leave many patients without adequate alternative care, given that outpatient services are quite limited.

2 Outpatient care. Outpatient care encompasses all care that is provided in a setting outside the hospital. It can come in the form of a standalone psychiatric clinic, as

part of a polyclinic (i.e. a clinic where a variety of diseases are treated by different specialists), attached to a hospital or a day treatment facility. As is to be expected, outpatient care is stratified similarly to inpatient care, with LICs providing the lowest availability and UMICs the highest. LICs had a median of 341 outpatient contacts per 100,000 population per year while UMICs had 5619 per 100,000 population per year (WHO 2009).

While clinics usually provide individual care to patients, day treatment facilities can deliver services to groups of patients. Patients participating in day treatment facilities typically spend several hours a day, up to five times a week, at the program, where they engage in group therapies, have their medications dispensed and are given the opportunity to socialize with peers. Many low income countries have no day treatment facilities, as these usually are indicators for a more developed mental health care system. While LICs have an average of 2.4 patients per 100,000 population utilizing this service, UMICs have an almost ten-fold proportion of patients (20.8/100,000 population) in day treatment facilities (WHO 2009).

3   Community outreach. Community outreach is considered part of outpatient-based care, where the providers actively seek out patients in the community and treat them in situ. Given that many developing countries lack proper infrastructure and transportation, a mental health mobile team can provide invaluable services to a community. Our experiences with mobile health teams have shown that they are generally well accepted within the community and can deliver fairly comprehensive and consistent care to homebound and geographically isolated patients.

4   Laws and policies. Any psychiatric care, whether inpatient or outpatient-based, is governed by the local laws and policies in place. Having a better understanding of these laws and policies will enable the global mental health professional to potentially effect positive change. Before expanding on the possible scenarios encountered, let us first describe the differences between mental health policies, action plans, and laws.

A mental health policy is a statement usually issued by a governmental authority that provides the direction for mental health care, while defining specific values and principles. It represents a best-case scenario vision of what a mental health program should encompass and includes statements about a country's mental health financing, legislation, organizational structure, treatment delivery, medication availability, and research, among others. A mental health action plan is the roadmap that details how a policy will be implemented. It lays out concretely each step necessary to complete the policy's vision. The WHO elegantly describes the relationship between policy and action plan as follows: 'A policy without strategic plan remains a dream. A plan without policy is an aimless and disorganized list of activities' (WHO 2007). Mental health legislation comprises a set of laws that codify the values of principles set forth in the mental health policy. Ideally, mental health law should protect the human rights of the mentally disabled and cover issues including access to treatment, quality of treatment, patient autonomy, and involuntary hospitalization.

Worldwide, a dedicated mental health policy exists in only 60 percent of countries. In low income countries this number drops to only about 50 percent.

Respectively, only 60 percent of all countries have mental health legislation, while only about 40 percent of LICs have mental health legislation (WHO 2011). One example of how the lack of policies or legislation can affect the care of patients is in the availability of psychotropic medications. McBain et al. (2012) describe how a mental health plan can increase the availability of psychotropic medication by 15 percent. There are numerous barriers that can affect the translation of legislation, policy, and plan into actual service delivery. Mental health tends to fall low on the list of financial priorities, likely because of a general lack of awareness and advocacy despite abundant stigma. The most comprehensive policy will not be implemented if sufficient funding is not allocated. We have seen this take place at one of our collaborative sites in the Caribbean where a complete mental health policy sat waiting for approval at the Ministry of Health for years. Furthermore, if necessary legislation is not in place, policy cannot be readily transformed into action.

5   Telepsychiatry: Telepsychiatry employs telecommunication technology, such as videoconferencing, to bring psychiatric services to remote areas. It can help connect non-psychiatrically trained staff and patients with clinicians in order to provide assessment and medication management as well as individual and group therapy. We will further discuss the benefits of telepsychiatry along with the significant barriers to its successful implementation in Chapter 11.

The following checklist should serve as a guide for assessing a community's non-human resources. Adhering to it will help illuminate a country's mental health care system's strengths and weaknesses and can provide ideas on how to implement change.

✓ Familiarize yourself with local mental health legislation and assess in what respect it is implemented or enforced.
✓ Familiarize yourself with local mental health policy and keep this in mind while assessing psychiatric services.
✓ Get to know the psychiatric services available (inpatient, outpatient, outreach, day treatment facilities, etc.) and pay attention to how easily they are accessed, not just by the local community, but also by surrounding communities.
✓ Acquaint yourself with available psychotropic medications and ask about consistency of availability, access, and cost.
✓ Ask about non-pharmacological treatment options, such as ECT, and how readily patients can access them.
✓ Inquire about and explore the infrastructure available to employ telepsychiatry.

After having discussed the human and non-human resources, we can begin to understand why Sam might not have been properly diagnosed. While he was able to access a primary care physician, this did not lead to the proper referral. Rather than pointing the finger at his primary care doctor, we should examine this missed opportunity from the perspective of a systemic failure. The doctor may not have considered depression as a cause for Sam's symptoms because of a lack of awareness or training, fortified by social stigma and local attitudes. Given that the psychiatric patients are 'locked away' at the mental health hospital, the doctor may have had virtually no experience in his education and training of properly diagnosing and treating psychiatric patients. His perception of the mentally ill is limited to the archaic concept of the 'insane' being housed in asylums, away from society. And how could this be any different given the resources available in his country? Without a system in place that addresses the specific needs of psychiatric patients, he would experience futility in recognizing mental illness among his patients. Furthermore, in order to increase his level of awareness, he would require training—training which in turn requires human and non-human resources: a collaborative professional that could teach him about mental health in primary care, access to textbooks, paper, or even a copy machine, to name a few.

References

Bauer, M., Adli, M., Bschor, T., Pilhatsch, M., Pfennig, A., Sasse, J., et al. 2010, 'Lithium's emerging role in the treatment of refractory major depressive episodes: augmentation of antidepressants,' *Neuropsychobiology*, vol. 62, no. 1, pp. 36–42.

Chanpattana, W., Kojima, K., Kramer, B.A., Intakorn, A., & Sasaki, S. 2005, 'ECT practice in Japan,' *The Journal of ECT*, vol. 21, no. 1, p. 58.

Chanpattana, W., Kramer, B.A., Kunigiri, G., Gangadhar, B., Kitphati, R., & Andrade, C. 2010, 'A survey of the practice of electroconvulsive therapy in Asia,' *The Journal of ECT*, vol. 26, no. 1, pp. 5–10.

Degenhardt, L., Whiteford, H.A., Ferrari, A.J., Baxter, A.J., Charlson, F.J., Hall, W.D., et al. 2013, 'Global burden of disease attributable to illicit drug use and dependence: findings from the Global Burden of Disease Study 2010,' *The Lancet*, vol. 382, no. 9904, pp. 1564–1574.

Hales, R., Yudofsky, S., & Weiss Roberts, L. 2014, 'Chapter 28. Brain stimulation therapies' in M. George, J. Taylor, E. Short, J. Snipes, & C. Pelic (eds.), *The American Psychiatric Publishing Textbook of Psychiatry*, 6th edn, American Psychiatric Publishing, Washington, DC.

Laing, R., Waning, B., Gray, A., Ford, N., & 't Hoen, E. 2003, '25 years of the WHO essential medicines lists: progress and challenges,' *The Lancet*, vol. 361, no. 9370, pp. 1723–1729.

Lakshmana, R., Hiscock, R., Galbally, M., Fung, A., Walker, S., Blankley, G., & Buist, A. 2014, 'Electroconvulsive therapy in pregnancy' in M. Galbally, M. Snellen, & A. Lewis (eds.), *Psychopharmacology and Pregnancy*, Springer, Berlin, Heidelberg, pp. 209–223.

Leiknes, K.A., Schweder, L.J., & Høie, B. 2012, 'Contemporary use and practice of electroconvulsive therapy worldwide,' *Brain and Behavior*, vol. 2, no. 3, pp. 283–344.

McBain, R., Norton, D.J., Morris, J., Yasamy, M.T., & Betancourt, T.S. 2012, 'The role of health systems factors in facilitating access to psychotropic medicines: a cross-sectional analysis of the WHO-AIMS in 63 low- and middle-income countries,' *PLoS Medicine*, vol. 9, no. 1, p. e1001166.

Nelson, A.I. 2005, 'A national survey of electroconvulsive therapy use in the Russian Federation,' *The Journal of ECT*, vol. 21, no. 3, pp. 151–157.

Patel, V., Minas, H., Cohen, A., & Prince, M. (eds.) 2014, *Global Mental Health, Principles and Practice*, 1st edn, Oxford University Press, New York.

Porter, R. 1999, *The Greatest Benefit To Mankind: A Medical History of Humanity*, 1st edn, W.W. Norton & Company, New York.

Prudic, J., Olfson, M., & Sackeim, H.A. 2001, 'Electro-convulsive therapy practices in the community,' *Psychological Medicine*, vol. 31, no. 05, pp. 929–934.

Schatzberg, A.F., Cole, J.O., & DeBattista, C. (eds.) 2010, *Manual of Clinical Psychopharmacology*, 7th edn, American Psychiatric Publishing, Arlington, VA.

van Schaik, A.M., Comijs, H.C., Sonnenberg, C.M., Beekman, A.T., Sienaert, P., & Stek, M.L. 2012, 'Efficacy and safety of continuation and maintenance electroconvulsive therapy in depressed elderly patients: a systematic review,' *The American Journal of Geriatric Psychiatry*, vol. 20, no. 1, pp. 5–17.

World Health Organization 1977, *The Selection of Essential Drugs: Report of a WHO Expert Committee*, World Health Organization, Geneva.

World Health Organization 2007, *Mental Health Policies and Action Plans: Key Issues and Basic Definitions*, World Health Organization, Geneva.

World Health Organization 2009, *Mental Health Systems in Selected Low- and Middle-income Countries: A WHO-AIMS Cross-national Analysis*, World Health Organization, Geneva.

World Health Organization 2011, *Mental Health Atlas 2011*, World Health Organization, Geneva.

World Health Organization 2014, *WHO Essential medicines*. Available: www.who.int/medicines/services/essmedicines_def/en/ (accessed January 19, 2014).

Chapter 4

Socioeconomic conditions

Imagine that, thanks to your successful integration into the 'system' and advocacy on behalf of mental health, you are invited to consult as a psychiatrist with Sam and his medical doctor. You conclude that Sam has major depressive disorder and prescribe the only antidepressant available, amitriptyline. He receives the prescription and is asked to return in two weeks. Sam's follow-up appointment comes and goes, but he does not appear. Instead he slipped back into his daily life . . .

Having only been educated up to the age of ten, Sam goes off to work on his rice farm ahead of the looming heat of the sun. His long tedious days are made tolerable by a local alcoholic beverage tapped from palm trees on the farm's perimeter. At day's end, he stops off at a street-side shack where men congregate on dusty milk crates to drink, eat a dinner of boiled rice, and play cards. For a while, though, he departed from his routine to attend a few rallies for a presidential candidate in hopes that they would bring more educational and employment opportunities to their country.

Sam eventually returns to an empty home lit by a battery powered flashlight perched in the doorway between its two rooms. His wife left long ago with their four school age children to live with her parents in a remote county far removed by a 10-hour journey from the center of the civil war. She also could no longer tolerate her husband's beatings. That he has not seen them in two years seems not to matter as Sam falls drunk onto the threadbare mat that is his bed, forgetting to take his amitriptyline.

The biopsychosocial approach to MH is a semantic and conceptual amalgam of the biological, psychological, and social dimensions that dictates that all possible contributors to someone's emotional wellbeing are taken account of (Engel 1977). It is a reminder to avoid over-emphasizing human psychology's impact on mental health. Instead, it underscores the contributions that our biological and social worlds play as well. Freud perhaps took it even further in famously writing, 'The human ego is first and foremost a bodily ego' (Freud 1923). And, in the end we can simplify things by saying that realities like Sam's are not to be overlooked.

When the global mental health professional steps off of the airplane and into the usually tropical host country, reality and the hot air usually greets them with a one-two slap. Especially in low income countries, the level of poverty can inject hopelessness into most ambitions, psychiatric or otherwise. So wrote one of our close colleagues about a line of thinking which dogged her while working on one of our collaborative psychiatric projects in West Africa:

> Mental Health experts could advocate for the mental well-being of individuals caught in a nonfunctional justice system. But is this psychiatry? What can all the 13 years of training in medical school, psychiatric residency, psychiatry geriatric fellowship followed by 5 years of work in a closely monitored top down, well-staffed, legally informed inpatient psychiatric unit with sophisticated tools for neuropsychiatric investigation, and social and psychological rehabilitative interventions at my disposal allow me to do for those suffering from emotional distress in settings where the causes are socio-political in nature?
>
> (Aloysi 2011a)

In this chapter, we will try to explore this uneasiness, as it is something that will confront any global mental health worker. It is also an issue that funders are sure to raise and should raise. We will review what the scientific literature has to say about the interaction between life circumstances and mental health. After that, we will talk about how we have to not just come to terms with lives like that of Sam but try to innovate in the face of it through the 'three A's'—attitude, advocacy, and activism.

Health, mental health, and living conditions

Health is determined by far more than health care (Woolf 2011). Social and economic conditions profoundly affect health. For example, educational and income levels both correlate with greater life expectancy (Woolf 2009). It has been suggested that physicians can and should step outside of their conventional biomedical approach to health and advocate for social changes as a route to better health. For example, since diabetics who graduate from college have lower diabetes related mortality than do high school graduates, might endocrinology societies advocate for educational reform as much as they do for precise insulin control (Woolf 2009)?

There is no reason to believe these same arguments could not be made about the relationship between socioeconomic conditions and psychiatry. If anything, psychiatry and its biopsychosocial tradition are predicated on this connection far more than any other field of medicine to such a degree that the connection seems intuitive. Perhaps for this reason there is only scattered, but revealing, literature on the subject. As the next section explores, the most abundant such literature involves financial security and wellbeing that appears to have been especially prompted by the worldwide 2008 economic downturn.

Financial security

Evidence supports how economic crises can impact on five elements of mental health—affective wellbeing, competence, autonomy, aspirations, and integrated functioning (Ng, Agius, & Zaman 2013). That is, the unemployed feel worse, experience a loss in self-confidence, feel less of a sense of control over their lives, lose hope for the future, and drop out of usual patterns of social involvement. Over a nearly 40-year period in Europe, unemployment correlated with increases in mortality from alcohol related deaths, violence, and also suicide in people less than 65 years of age (Stuckler et al. 2009). Domestic violence and child abuse likely increase in economic crises for a variety of interrelated reasons that certainly include alcohol use (Ng et al. 2013).

In the 'poverty trap', mental health problems beget poverty and poverty begets mental health problems (Manderscheid 2013). On the one hand, this notion suggests that conventional treatment of mental health problems can help to alleviate poverty by enhancing drive, hope, focus, confidence, and social involvement. On the other hand, active steps to address conditions of poverty can help to alleviate some mental health problems. The latter suggests that if mental health professionals truly care about the whole patient, they would consider addressing poverty like Sam's to be a professional responsibility.

It may be apparent that the data cited so far regarding financial security and mental health derives from the developed world, leading to the potential supposition that people who are unaccustomed to severe financial stress are less able to cope with it than those who do so on a regular basis. But, there is some evidence for this relationship as well from the developing world. A comprehensive review examining the evidence for the poverty trap in low and middle income countries found significant evidence that improvements in mental health do beget reductions in poverty (but did not find a significant effect of poverty alleviation on mental health) (Lund et al. 2011). The study authors declared that scaling up mental health services should therefore be considered a development priority. Among urban dwellers in West Africa's Ghana and in a manner reminiscent of Sam, low income, low education, large family size, difficult life events ('hard times'), and working in agriculture were all associated with psychological distress (Dzator 2013). Maintaining non-agricultural employment through hard times was felt to be psychologically protective and an important focus for public planners.

Figure 4.1 shows a composite look at the relationship of health, mental health, and economic crisis.

Food security

Food insecurity and mental health have also been found to be interrelated. In a US study of adolescents, low socioeconomic status correlated with food insecurity, which in turn increased the chances of having had a mood, anxiety, or substance use disorder in the last year. This effect was independent of poverty level (McLaughlin et al. 2012). When we shift across the world to rural Tanzania in Africa, food insecurity in women caretakers in four different ethnic groups was highly correlated with scores of clinical anxiety and depression (Hadley & Patil 2006). The authors of that study suggested that determining the direction of causality in this relationship has less relevance than finding solutions to the larger societal issues that foster these problems such as marginalization of women from the mainstream economy (Hadley & Patil 2006). Finally, a quantifiable threshold has been found

Reduced Tax Revenue
- Lower government spending on health – immunization, health insurance, R&D
- Lower government spending on education, subsidies, and transfers

Economic Crisis
- Reduced economic growth rates
- Higher unemployment & under-employment
- Higher inflation
- Higher bankruptcy rates

Reduced Health Status
- Mortality rates
- Increased mental health cases
- Increased prevalence of malnutrition & wasting
- Life expectancy

Reduced Household Real Income
- Low quality & quantity of food
- Reduced resources for health care
- Lower school retention rates
- Reduced carer services as more care givers join workforce to supplement income
- Increased crime
- Family breakdowns

Figure 4.1 Relationship between economic crisis and health status

Source: Dzator 2013

beyond which spikes in food prices appear to have provoked mass social unrest in countries in North Africa and the Middle East (Lagi, Bertrand, & Bar-Yam 2011).

Climate

There may also be a relationship between extreme temperatures and mental health issues. Mental health is adversely affected by fuel insecurity and 'cold housing' across all age groups. For example, adolescents living in cold houses have a 1 in 4 risk of developing mental illness compared to a 1 in 20 risk in those who always have a warm home (Marmot Review Team 2011). At the other extreme reminiscent of Sam's hot toiling in the rice fields, rising temperatures related to climate change are predicted to cause reductions in work productivity and heightened work stress among outdoor workers in low and middle income countries (Kjellstrom, Holmer, & Lemke 2009). This impact should be modifiable via changes to the outdoor workplace. Meanwhile, direct and indirect connections exist between climate change and mental health conditions. The former could result from the direct trauma of extreme weather events as well as elevated aggression and suicidality from extreme temperatures in particular. Climate change can indirectly affect mental health via its influence over physical health as well as its destabilizing effects on the living environment (Berry, Bowen, & Kjellstrom 2010).

Social advocacy and activism

> [H]ealth officials, organized medicine, disease-related groups, care delivery systems, and academia must embrace the tenet that social change is a legitimate tool for improving health.
>
> (Woolf 2009)

To this list we add global mental health professionals. In the face of countless situations like Sam's across the world, focusing on the psychological or biological aspects of his depressive disorder to the exclusion of the social ones may be pragmatic and may be most in line with our training and our bent, but it is shortsighted. Most mental health professionals will reflexively acknowledge the important contribution life circumstances make to people's emotional wellbeing. As we alluded to earlier, this verges on being so intuitive as to be a truism for anyone who stops to think about it. However, in global mental health practice perhaps more so than elsewhere in the field of mental health, we need to go beyond dutifully acknowledging the connection between socioeconomic circumstances to embracing it. There are three progressively more engaged paths for accomplishing this—*attitude, advocacy, and activism.*

Attitude

An attitude of social-mindedness is essential to the mindset of anyone participating in global mental health practice—health, mental health, and allied health professionals or collaborators in community and government. Like traveling to someone's country to be with them in body, it entails going to where they are to be with them in spirit. In practice, such an attitude involves acknowledging it to oneself and acknowledging it to one's hosts by finding an empathic middle ground that avoids condescension.

This middle ground is situated atop one of two messages: (1) *Modest*—'I am learning how rough things are here and will do my own small part with the mental health tools I have to help you and your community cope the best you can'; or (2) *Ambitious*—'I am learning how rough things are here and am prepared to do what I can and work with who I can to help you and your community try to change things for the better.' Assuming one of these positions helps to accomplish two things. Intangibly speaking, it will help the global mental health practitioner gain acceptance in a community in which they are otherwise an outsider. Practically speaking, it will broadly help set a course of action.

For example, while we were involved in a mental health needs assessment trip to the 2004 South Asian Tsunami in Sri Lanka about a month after the event, we encountered a staggering loss of life and property. What Sri Lankans most needed to feel better was the impossibility of somehow again being with those family and friends they had lost to the sea. At the least, getting back their homes and their livelihoods (often as fishermen) would suffice under the circumstances. It was oppressively humbling to hear a gentleman kneeling under a tree with friends say: 'I lost my wife and daughter, my home, my boat, and even the clothes off of my back. What is there for me?'

Not having ever before worked as mental health professionals in Sri Lanka and with only one of us being a native Sri Lankan who had herself not lived there in years, neither our expertise nor our professional relationships positioned us to adopt the *ambitious* attitude of trying to help people get back their homes and jobs. We adopted a *modest* attitude and asked our new colleagues there in the health and business sectors, especially the Rotary Clubs who were our hosts, how we could best deploy our mental health expertise in the name of their country's recovery. The answer was to help train the equivalent of community mental health workers and even some interested business people to be lay mental health counselors by sharing and 'translating' what we knew about post-disaster adult and child mental health needs and interventions (see also Chapter 9).

Advocacy

By *advocacy* we mean working on behalf of an individual with an identified mental health problem to address some element of their social circumstances that is assessed to be clinically relevant. Advocacy is one outgrowth of an *ambitious* attitude. In usual practice in the developed world, this often means referring them to a social worker. In global mental health practice, this may be an option, especially if there is a Ministry of Social Welfare with which to work. Where possible, partnering with them would greatly maximize the potential benefit of global mental health programming beyond traditional consultation room based treatment. Often local social workers have access to distressingly limited resources and benefits, but they still have more knowledge and access than even a visiting social worker practicing in global mental health would be starting with.

On the other hand, local social workers may be in short supply, leaving the global mental health professional or a global mental health program to decide whether they have the ability, energy, and time to go beyond prescribing antidepressants to address 'concrete needs.' Here, the global mental health professional or program can become the 'Swiss Army knife' described elsewhere in this book. Indeed, it is a virtue of having a multi-disciplinary global mental health approach that social service needs could be addressed by an appropriately trained and tasked member of that team such as a visiting social worker.

In Sam's case, the advocacy opportunities run the gamut. It is not clear that he prioritizes re-uniting with his family but if he did or it was deemed prudent to encourage him to do so, even helping to facilitate a phone call or visit to his wife and kids would be a start. Providing him with money or a phone to do so could provide the spark that that sets good things in motion for him and them. In parallel with this would need to be involving him with a domestic violence program if one exists or providing him with counseling about domestic violence as well as drinking. Another big picture item for advocacy might be finding out if and how he could further his education through activities of governmental or non-governmental organizations (NGO).

At the smallest level, the advocate could buy Sam another flashlight and batteries so he has one for each room—a small but relatively sustainable social intervention. Indeed, a creative intervention would supply him with batteries at a monthly visit to the doctor or psychiatrist back in the capital. Such incentivized visits would simultaneously permit them to check on the progress of his clinical depression and the status of his amitriptyline prescription.

Activism

Activism by the global mental health professional involves systems level advocacy to change something that has broad impact on the mental health of people throughout a community. With the right assessment of a community's needs, this means 'bumping' up advocacy efforts to the community level and represents the other expression of an *ambitious* attitude. From Sam's example, it might entail working to bring an education oriented NGO into his village or region or to at least bring Sam's village to their attention. If Sam's undetected problem with alcohol reflects a community wide issue, setting up alcohol self-help groups on a village-by-village basis might be on target. It might even mean raising money to purchase flashlights for an entire village.

One example of global mental health activism at perhaps the highest level involves the elimination of unmodified ECT (i.e., electro-convulsive therapy done without anesthesia; see Chapter 3 for more details) in Turkey (Aloysi 2011b). In 2006, the group Mental Health Disability Rights International published a report detailing human rights abuses in Turkey's psychiatric hospitals. This led the largest psychiatric hospital in Turkey to replace its director with a new psychiatrist who within a few months eliminated the use of unmodified ECT at that facility. Meanwhile, the Turkish government agreed to eliminate unmodified ECT across the country by assigning anesthesiologists to all psychiatric hospitals.

While the example from Turkey is admittedly activism within the realm of mental health policy, we also encourage global mental health professionals to consider thinking (we might even say dreaming) 'outside the box' in order to potentially maximize their mental health impact on the world. In Liberia, where we have observed countless cases of childhood cerebral malaria leading to a lifetime of cognitive, emotional, and behavioral sequelae for those children who survive the acute illness, a vital mental health oriented project that remains to be done is a formal study of the extent of the problem along with an analysis of the modifiable risk factors and potential early interventions that could reduce the incidence of this problem (Mishra & Newton 2009). Would better provision of insecticide treated mosquito nets have a far greater public health and mental health impact for the Liberians than reactively trying to supply the country with psychotropic medications and related therapies to treat cerebral malaria survivors? And, instead of focusing on provision of specialized psychiatric care, would an educational campaign explaining the reason these children behave as they do de-stigmatize the situation enough that they are welcomed into schools more and shunned less by playmates?

We especially encourage consideration of using work rehabilitation programs to help de-compress overcrowded psychiatric hospitals of the chronic mentally ill. Evidence suggests they can improve psychiatric symptoms and prevent re-hospitalization for many patients (Reker & Eikelmann 1997). Their benefits surely derive from the sense of purpose, socializing, and income they can afford the mentally ill as does the right work for anyone. As such, they may address psychological distress as well as financial distress and provide a way to address both sides of the 'poverty trap.'

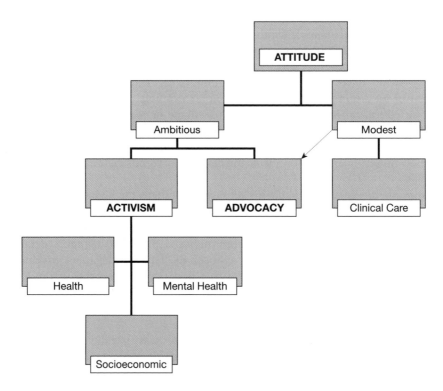

Figure 4.2 The three A's of socioeconomic involvement

Conclusions

Ultimately, it is not the case that people's life circumstances are more or less of an important consideration than their mental health but rather that addressing them is not an either-or proposition. And, we believe that global mental health professionals can become advocates or activists for social change that can drive people towards better mental health as much as mental health can drive social change. However, we do not suggest that all global mental health professionals must become advocates or activists.

As reflected in Figure 4.2, we do believe that the minimal requirement for being a global mental health worker is a socioeconomically oriented attitude towards mental health issues. There is a considerable likelihood that if you are reading this book, you are already self-selected for this attitude. Either way, we have attempted to build on this by providing you with a systematic way to both personally and professionally deal with the harsh dose of reality we inevitably encounter in working in low and middle income countries and other low resource settings. The '3 A's' framework is our response to our colleague's pangs of grave self-doubt while working in West Africa. It should ideally permit you to function and feel at your best in global mental health work by helping you to articulate a vision of your biopsychosocial self or program for yourself, your colleagues, and those you intend to help.

We recommend that you employ Figure 4.2 as a 'socioeconomic checklist' for yourself as you prepare for your global mental health work. You should then be open to re-assessing it while in the field, possibly more than once and in discussion with colleagues and hosts. And you should decide how much you fulfilled your checklist when your travel ends. It should help you to appreciate what work remains to be done and how it can realistically continue if not on future trips then from afar. As one of our close colleagues in the Eastern Caribbean often reminds us, any contribution you make to the mental health of a community counts.

References

Aloysi, A. 2011a, *Reflections on Liberia*, unpublished personal journal.

Aloysi, A.S. 2011b, *Barriers to the Provision of Modified Electroconvulsive Therapy in Resource-Poor Settings*, Mount Sinai School of Medicine, New York.

Berry, H.L., Bowen, K., & Kjellstrom, T. 2010, 'Climate change and mental health: a causal pathways framework,' *International Journal of Public Health*, vol. 55, no. 2, pp. 123–132.

Dzator, J. 2013, 'Hard times and common mental health disorders in developing countries: insights from urban Ghana,' *The Journal of Behavioral Health Services & Research*, vol. 40, no. 1, pp. 71–87.

Engel, G.L. 1977, 'The need for a new medical model: a challenge for biomedicine,' *Science*, vol. 196, no. 4286, pp. 129–136.

Freud, S. 1923, 'The Ego and the Id' in *The Ego and the Id and Other Works* (ed. J. Strachey), Hogarth Press, London, pp. 1–66.

Hadley, C. & Patil, C.L. 2006, 'Food insecurity in rural Tanzania is associated with maternal anxiety and depression,' *American Journal of Human Biology*, vol. 18, no. 3, pp. 359–368.

Kjellstrom, T., Holmer, I., & Lemke, B. 2009, 'Workplace heat stress, health and productivity—an increasing challenge for low and middle-income countries during climate change,' *Global Health Action*, vol. 2, pp. 1–6.

Lagi, M., Bertrand, K., & Bar-Yam, Y. 2011, *The Food Crises and Political Instability in North Africa and the Middle East*. Available: arxiv.org/pdf/1108.2455 (accessed December 15, 2014).

Lund, C., De Silva, M., Plagerson, S., Cooper, S., Chisholm, D., Das, J., et al. 2011, 'Poverty and mental disorders: breaking the cycle in low-income and middle-income countries,' *Lancet*, vol. 378, no. 9801, pp. 1502–1514.

Manderscheid, R. 2013, 'Escaping the "poverty trap",' *Behavioral Healthcare*, vol. 33, no. 4, pp. 49–50.

Marmot Review Team 2011, *The Health Impacts of Cold Homes and Fuel Poverty*, Friends of the Earth and Marmor Review Team, London.

McLaughlin, K.A., Green, J.G., Alegria, M., Jane Costello, E., Gruber, M.J., Sampson, N.A., & Kessler, R.C. 2012, 'Food insecurity and mental disorders in a national sample of U.S. adolescents,' *Journal of the American Academy of Child and Adolescent Psychiatry*, vol. 51, no. 12, pp. 1293–1303.

Mishra, S.K. & Newton, C.R. 2009, 'Diagnosis and management of the neurological complications of falciparum malaria,' *Nature Reviews Neurology*, vol. 5, no. 4, pp. 189–198.

Ng, K.H., Agius, M., & Zaman, R. 2013, 'The global economic crisis: effects on mental health and what can be done,' *Journal of the Royal Society of Medicine*, vol. 106, no. 6, pp. 211–214.

Reker, T. & Eikelmann, B. 1997, 'Work therapy for schizophrenic patients: results of a 3-year prospective study in Germany,' *European Archives of Psychiatry and Clinical Neuroscience,* vol. 247, no. 6, pp. 314–319.

Stuckler, D., Basu, S., Suhrcke, M., Coutts, A., & McKee, M. 2009, 'The public health effect of economic crises and alternative policy responses in Europe: an empirical analysis,' *The Lancet,* vol. 374, no. 9686, pp. 315–323.

Woolf, S.H. 2009, 'Social policy as health policy,' *JAMA: The Journal of the American Medical Association,* vol. 301, no. 11, pp. 1166–1169.

Woolf, S.H. 2011, 'Public health implications of government spending reductions,' *JAMA: The Journal of the American Medical Association,* vol. 305, no. 18, pp. 1902–1903.

Part 2

Clinical interventions

Chapter 5

Pharmacology

Unpacking the new shipment of amitriptyline, George receives a phone call from a psychiatrist working at the mental hospital outside of town. He is one of only two psychiatrists in the country and has been tasked with taking care of the several hundred inpatients admitted to the overcrowded and understaffed facility. Many of the chronic patients have been there for years and will likely never leave due to the absence of residential facilities or other intensive outpatient treatment options.

The psychiatrist calls to ask George about the availability of antidepressants. Just as George is about to eagerly tell him of his new shipment, the psychiatrist elaborates on his particular request: he would like a specific antidepressant, venlafaxine. A 57-year-old woman has been admitted to the hospital for severe depression and suicidality. She is a native who recently returned from the US, where she had gone to live with an aunt in the hopes of getting better psychiatric care for her chronic depression. After the death of her aunt she could no longer afford to stay in the US and flew back home with enough medication to last a few weeks. She ran out of her medication, venlafaxine, one of the only medications that has proven efficacious for her, and became increasingly depressed.

Frustrated by his inability to help in this situation, George notifies the doctor that venlafaxine is not available through his pharmacy. It is not one of the 'essential medicines' that the Ministry of Health provides access to. He suggests amitriptyline, he has plenty of it and the availability should be fairly guaranteed for the next month or so. He also suggests ordering venlafaxine from the local private pharmacy, if the patient is willing to pay for it.

Up until the development of chlorpromazine and the first tricyclic antidepressants in the 1950s, psychiatric treatment was limited to psychotherapeutic interventions, ECT, other convulsive therapies, and horrifying psychosurgeries. Being a psychiatric patient meant having to endure invasive treatments, at times torturous in nature, or a significant loss of freedom from lengthy hospitalizations (Shorter 1997). The development of psychiatric medications meant patients could be treated in the community and could therefore lead fuller and more productive lives. Over the years new agents have been developed, with fewer side effects, broader therapeutic windows, and lower toxicity (Baldessarini 2013).

The WHO Model List of Essential Medicines (MLEM) was briefly reviewed in Chapter 3 as playing a role in the non-human resources that comprise mental health care. Here we will take a closer look at the list by exploring the history of inclusion of psychotropic medications as well as the actual implementation and adherence of countries to it. We will also take a look at the data describing how vast a psychotropic armamentarium is needed to cover most major mental illnesses and compare this with the WHO list. Next, we will examine some cross-cultural considerations in using psychotropic medications, highlighting how race can influence metabolism as well as how attitudes towards medications may vary depending on the environment.

Finally, we invite the reader to consider the scenario above and ask how these circumstances would affect the way they might deliver psychiatric care and their choice of pharmacological intervention. We will explore the different scenarios and offer some perspectives on how to effectively navigate such dilemmas.

WHO Model Lists of Essential Medicines

History

Advances in medicine during the 20th century revolutionized the way health care was provided. One of the greatest milestones was the discovery and development of effective medicines, starting with penicillin in 1928. It was not until the 1940s that penicillin was effectively implemented and used to treat a wider patient population (Quirke 2001). That decade also saw the introduction of other revolutionizing medications such as the first anti-tuberculosis drug, streptomycin, as well as the first commercially available and well-tolerated anti-malarial, chloroquine (Sacks & Behrman 2008, Krafts, Hempelmann, & Skórska-Stania 2012). Within only a few years, physicians were suddenly able to effectively treat several infectious diseases that were a major contributor to the global burden of disease. The following decades were no less instrumental in lowering the world's burden of disease as they represented a major improvement in the development of medicines to treat non-communicable diseases, such as diabetes, cardiovascular disease, cancer, and psychiatric conditions.

Interestingly, the discovery of the first antipsychotic medication, chlorpromazine, grew out of research dedicated to anti-malarial compounds. As has often been the case with discovery, it was a string of coincidences and astute observations that led researchers to that conclusion. Efforts to find an alternative, less toxic medication to treat malaria led to the development of phenothiazines. This class of drugs was found to show greater efficacy as an antihistamine than an anti-malarial and was therefore used as a sedative. Agitated psychiatric patients who were given chlorpromazine not only became sedated shortly after administration, but their overall symptoms of psychosis seemed to greatly improve as well. This discovery revolutionized the way psychiatrists could treat psychotic illness and changed the landscape of psychiatric treatment forever (Shen 1999). By the late 1950s, psychiatric hospitalizations had significantly decreased worldwide and continued to do so for the rest of the century (Thullier 1999).

By the 1970s the pharmaceutical industry had developed medications to treat most major illnesses. Although many of these medications were not considered highly efficacious, they did offer treatment and hope to patients who had access to them (Baldessarini 2013). Yet all of these advances and breakthroughs had little to no impact in over half of the world's population, as medications were not readily available or affordable. Many developing countries had been decolonized over the past decades and were in desperate need to modernize their health care. As far as they were concerned, much of their medical care remained at the level of the early 20th century.

The WHO sought to change these global circumstances in 1975 by introducing the concept of essential medicines during its annual World Health Assembly meeting. This meeting represented a watershed in the way medicine availability would be conceived moving forward. The WHO introduced the idea of the *essential medicine*, with the goal of filling the gap between the potential of modern medicines and the limited capability of developing countries to utilize them, by influencing domestic policy (Reich 1987). This gap was the result of multiple factors, including lack of financial resources, irresponsible business practices of the pharmaceutical industry, inadequate social infrastructure leading to procurement and implementation difficulties as well as lack of facilities to assess drug quality (Reich 1987).

According to the WHO, essential medicines were considered 'to be of the utmost importance and hence basic, indispensable, and necessary for the health needs of the population. They should be available at all times, in the proper dosage forms, to all segments of society' (Resolution 1975). In 1977 the WHO published the first model list of essential medicines along with guidelines for countries on how to create their own list (WHO 1977). This list was intended to represent an example of an affordable yet comprehensive formulary that could be adopted by developing countries. Given that every country faces their own set of health problems, countries were encouraged to identify their priorities and customize their list accordingly. In addition to providing a model list, the WHO also initiated a widespread discussion about national drug policy, which continues to influence countries today. National drug policy, a concept that had not been part of the global health discussion prior to 1975, is described as:

> a commitment to a goal and a guide for action. It expresses and prioritizes the medium- to long-term goals set by the government for the pharmaceutical sector, and identifies the main strategies for attaining them. It provides a framework within which the activities of the pharmaceutical sector can be coordinated.
>
> (World Health Organization 2001)

Its main objectives are, simply put, to improve access to medications, as well as ensure their quality and rational use by influencing both the public and private sector.

The WHO's efforts have led to significant improvements in medication availability across the world. While only a handful of countries had national drug policies in 1975, 108 countries had adopted a national drug policy by the late 1990s (Creese et al. 2004). Similarly, access to medications has greatly improved since then, though it remains a hurdle in developing low and middle income countries.

Inclusion of medicines

The WHO Expert Committee on Selection and Use of Essential Medicines meets every two years to review the latest scientific evidence on the efficacy, safety, and cost effectiveness of medications in the MLEM. Applications for inclusion of medications can be submitted to the WHO by anyone, as long as they are complete and submitted four months prior to the Expert Committee Meeting. Two Committee members review all the applications and invite comments by leading specialists and organizations. Finally, the full Committee meets to revise the completed list before passing it on to the Director General of the WHO for final approval (WHO 2014).

Psychotropic medications

The first publication of the WHO Model List of Essential Medicines (WHO 1977) included six psychotropic medications:

- Chlorpromazine
- Haloperidol
- Fluphenazine
- Amitriptyline
- Lithium
- Diazepam.

Over the years, the amount of psychotropics in the core list has doubled and currently comprises those shown in Table 5.1.

Table 5.1 Current psychotropic medications within the WHO Model List of Essential Medicines, 18th edition

Medicines used in psychotic disorders
Chlorpromazine Fluphenazine Haloperidol Risperidone
Medicines used in depressive disorders
Amitriptyline Fluoxetine
Medicines used in bipolar disorders
Carbamazepine Lithium carbonate Valproic acid (sodium valproate)
Medicines for anxiety disorders
Diazepam
Medicines used for obsessive compulsive disorders
Clomipramine
Medicines for disorders due to psychoactive substance use
Nicotine replacement therapy (NRT) Methadone

Of note, while not specifically listed in the category of medicines for behavioral disorders, biperiden is also on the current list of essential medicines. Biperiden is an anti-parkinsonism drug that can effectively treat extrapyramidal side-effects of antipsychotic medications and should be considered as part of the psychiatric practitioner's formulary (Stanilla & Simpson 2009).

Discussion of current psychotropics included in the MLEM

While the MLEM is in no way comprehensive, it does provide the psychiatric practitioner with a fairly decent armamentarium of medications to treat various psychiatric illnesses. The following is a discussion of the scenario a mental health practitioner might encounter assuming a country or community has ongoing access to these essential medications along with practitioners who skillfully can implement them. We will also comment on what medications that are currently not on the MLEM would be needed to further enhance this armamentarium.

- Psychotic disorders
    - o In our experience patients with psychotic disorders stand a very good chance of receiving appropriate treatment and the practitioner can expect to see significant improvement. Provided there is access to anticholinergic medications such as benztropine, trihexylphenidyl, or biperiden (listed on the current MLEM), practitioners can expect to effectively minimize the side effects particular to antipsychotic medications (extrapyramidal side effects or EPS) (Stanilla & Simpson 2009). Clozapine, an antipsychotic with good efficacy in treatment-resistant cases listed on the complementary list, requires weekly blood monitoring. Access to a laboratory that can run basic blood tests (complete blood count) would therefore open the door for use of this medication (Marder & Wirshing 2009). With access to the above listed medications, a wide range of patients could be treated. Hence, no further additions to the list would be deemed necessary.

- Depressive disorders
    - o Patients with depressive disorders who have access to either amitriptyline or fluoxetine will have a fairly good chance of showing improvement, provided they receive uninterrupted treatment for several weeks to months (Nelson 2009; Zahajszky, Rosenbaum, & Tollefson 2009). However, more complex and treatment refractory cases may be difficult to treat with only these two drugs. The practitioner could try to augment with lithium or risperidone and likely effect some improvement (Freeman, Wiegand, & Gelenberg 2009; Goff 2009). The addition of a few other antidepressants from different classes (such as venlafaxine, bupropion, and mirtazapine) to the local formulary would provide more comprehensive treatment options, especially in regards to minimizing side effects (Thase & Sloan 200; Clayton & Gillespie 2009; Schatzberg 2009).

- Bipolar disorder
    - o Lithium and valproic acid are excellent first-choice medications to manage acute mania in bipolar disorder as well as preventing further manic episodes

(Freeman et al. 2009; Kemp et al. 2009). Medications from the class of anti-psychotics further complement the practitioner's toolbox for treating bipolar disorder, especially when the mania is accompanied by psychosis (Schatzberg, Cole, & DeBattista 2010). We would therefore consider that a majority of patients with bipolar disorder, who present with manic episodes, could be effectively treated with the above-mentioned essential medicines. Patients suffering mostly from bipolar depression are less likely to respond to the above medications and therefore would require the careful addition of an antidepressant (both amitriptyline and fluoxetine could be used) (Schatzberg et al. 2010). One medication that is not on the MLEM, which shows fairly good efficacy in treating and preventing bipolar depression, is lamotrigine (Kemp et al. 2009). Given its side effect risk profile, especially after stopping and restarting (which is often the case with only intermittently available drugs), it will not likely become an essential medicine. However, with ensured continuous availability this medication could nicely round out the formulary for bipolar disorder.

- Anxiety disorders

    o Diazepam is considered a good all-round medication to treat acute anxiety states. For the treatment of chronic anxiety and panic disorder, fluoxetine or amitriptyline may be preferred as they do not lead to dependence and the side effects from abrupt discontinuation are less concerning. As discussed in Chapter 3, diazepam further has the benefit of being highly effective to treat seizures and can be used to treat insomnia, alcohol withdrawal, and muscle spasms (Sheehan & Raj 2009). With diazepam, fluoxetine, and amitriptyline we would expect to be able to treat a fairly large number of patients for anxiety with good results (Sheehan & Raj 2009; Zahajszky, Rosenbaum, & Tollefson 2009; Nelson 2009). A more comprehensive formulary may include the addition of shorter acting anti-anxiety drugs such as lorazepam or alprazolam (Sheehan & Raj 2009).

    o Patients with obsessive-compulsive disorder (OCD) are somewhat less likely to receive sufficient treatment. While clomipramine is well suited, it can cause undesirable side effects, such as sedation, dry mouth, blurry vision, or consti-pation (Nelson 2009). Fluoxetine can also be utilized to treat OCD (Zahajszky et al. 2009). The availability of fluvoxamine would provide the practitioner with an additional solid tool to treat these patients while minimizing side effects.

- Substance abuse disorders

    o Opioid dependence is a large contributor to morbidity worldwide (Degenhardt et al. 2013) and therefore requires adequate attention. While methadone is listed in the complementary MLEM, it has in our experience not been a readily available drug in developing countries. Buprenorphine, another very effective medicine used to treat opioid addiction (Schatzberg et al. 2010) is also mentioned in the complementary list as an additional medication in this class. Assuming a practitioner had access to these two medications, he or she would be able to treat a majority of opioid dependent patients, provided the right infrastructure were available. Comprehensive substance abuse treatment should always include the availability of self-help groups as well as individual and group counseling.

o   Alcohol use disorder, a huge contributor to the global burden of disease (Whiteford et al. 2013), can also be treated with medications. As with the treatment of other substance use disorders, embedding pharmacotherapy in a comprehensive framework leads to greater success. We have found that despite the rampant prevalence of alcohol use disorders worldwide, few developing countries are adequately equipped to treat this condition. The issue most commonly addressed is alcohol *withdrawal*, which can be successfully treated using the essential medicines diazepam or valproic acid (Sheehan & Raj 2009; Bowden 2009). While we suggest having the following medications at one's disposal, it should be understood that their successful implementation is largely dependent on treatment infrastructure: Disulfiram is a drug used to create an unpleasant bodily reaction when individuals use alcohol (Schatzberg et al. 2010). It requires individuals to be highly motivated and disciplined. Acamprosate helps reduce cravings, but has been shown to be most effective when combined with counseling services. Naltrexone can also be used to treat cravings and reduce the rewarding effects of alcohol (Schatzberg et al. 2010). The practitioner who has some or all of these medicines at his or her disposal should therefore make every effort to integrate his or her patients into a structured treatment framework.

- Additional medications needed

o   While the MLEM does address dosing considerations for the child and adolescent population, it nonetheless misses out on the treatment of a major contributor to childhood morbidity: attention deficit-hyperactivity disorder (ADHD), which is estimated to be prevalent in about 6 percent of school age children (Polanczyk et al. 2007). In our view, the exclusion of stimulants such as methylphenidate from the MLEM has created a significant treatment gap in children and adolescents. Multiple studies have shown that early treatment of childhood ADHD leads to significant improvements in overall functioning later in life as well as a reduction of risk of substance abuse (Biederman 2003; Wilens et al. 2003; Shaw et al. 2012). None of the countries we have worked in carry stimulants on their national formulary and these patients generally do not receive appropriate care, despite ever-increasing referrals from pediatricians and general practitioners. A well-rounded psychotropic armamentarium should therefore include at least one stimulant, such as methylphenidate.

In order to understand the influence of the WHO MLEM on individual countries, we will compare its psychotropics to the essential medicine lists of five countries we have worked in, Belize, Haiti, Liberia, India, and St Vincent and the Grenadines (SVG) (see Table 5.2).

Of the countries listed, Belize has by far the largest formulary, which is consistent with its fairly well developed mental health program. Most countries evidently structure their formulary based on the WHO, with most additions being older (and subsequently inexpensive) medicines. Note, as mentioned above, that none of the

Table 5.2 WHO Model List of Essential Medicines compared to five developing countries' essential medicine lists

WHO[1]	Belize[2]	Haiti[3]	India[4]	Liberia[5]	SVG[6]
Psychotic disorders					
Chlorpromazine	Chlorpromazine	Chlorpromazine	Chlorpromazine	Chlorpromazine	Chlorpromazine
Fluphenazine	Fluphenazine	Fluphenazine		Fluphenazine	Fluphenazine
Haloperidol	Haloperidol	Haloperidol	Haloperidol	Haloperidol	Haloperidol
	Thioridazine				Thioridazine
	Flupenthixol				
	Trifluperazine				Trifluperazine
				Benzhexol	
Risperidone[7]	Risperidone			Risperidone	
	Quetiapine		Olanzapine		
Complementary list					
Clozapine[7]	Clozapine				Risperdal
					Zuclopenthixol
Depressive disorders					
Amitriptyline	Amitriptyline	Amitriptyline	Amitriptyline	Amitriptyline	Amitriptyline
Fluoxetine	Fluoxetine		Fluoxetine	Fluoxetine	Fluoxetine
	Sertraline				
	Imipramine		Imipramine		Imipramine
Bipolar disorders					
Carbamazepine	Carbamazepine	Carbamazepine		Carbamazepine	Carbamazepine
Lithium	Lithium	Lithium	Lithium	Lithium	Lithium
Valproic acid	Valproic acid		Valproic acid	Valproic acid	Valproic acid

Anxiety disorders	Diazepam	Diazepam Clonazepam Lorazepam Alprazolam	Diazepam	Diazepam Alprazolam	Diazepam	Diazepam
OCD	Clomipramine	Clomipramine	Clomipramine	Fluoxetine	Clomipramine	Clomipramine
Substance use disorders	Nicotine replacement Methadone	Methadone			Methadone Buprenorphine	Methadone

Notes:
1 WHO Model List of Essential Medicines, 18th Edition, 2013
2 Belize Drug Formulary, 9th Edition, 2009–2011
3 Haiti Liste Nationale Des Médicaments Essentiels, 1st Edition, 2012
4 National List of Essential Medicines of India, 3rd Edition, 2011
5 Liberia Essential Medicine List, 2nd Edition, 2011
6 St. Vincent and the Grenadines Essential Medicine List, 1st Edition 2010
7 Added to WHO MLEM in 2013

countries list stimulants as essential medicines and therefore do not carry them in their government-funded pharmacies. While Liberia and SVG have listed methadone as an essential medicine, we have not found this medication to be locally available. Also, note that there are no medicines available to treat alcohol use disorder despite the pervasively high prevalence of this condition.

Cross-cultural considerations

When practitioners prescribe medications, regardless of the type, there are numerous factors that can and should be considered. For starters, will the medication be effective? Will the patient take it correctly? Will they take it at all? Can he or she afford to buy it? What does it mean for the patient to receive (or not receive) a prescription? How does their cultural/ethnic/racial background affect how willing they are to take this medication? And does their background affect how efficacious the medication will be or whether they are more/less likely to encounter side effects?

These are questions that prescribers should ask themselves, regardless if they practice in a high or low income country. The latter questions become progressively important as migration has increased over the last century and our populations grow ever more heterogeneous. Global mental health practitioners working in a resource-scarce community should equip themselves with the knowledge needed to answer these questions. Doing so will greatly enhance the impact one can make. Here we will look at how ethnicity and race interact with pharmacotherapy.

Attitudes towards psychiatric medications

A person's willingness to take psychotropic medications depends first and foremost on their conceptualization of mental illness. A condition that is generally not considered to be 'an illness' will not prompt the search for a remedy. Cross-cultural studies show that psychotic disorders are almost universally considered mental illnesses, though the etiology varies. A common explanation for a person developing psychosis, one that we have encountered ourselves on numerous occasions, is that of being possessed by a (possibly evil) spirit. Patients and their families will consequently seek out treatment from traditional healers, though often in conjunction with medical professionals. Depression on the other hand is often not identified as a mental illness or a condition requiring treatment at all, and hence is not treated.

Attitudes towards medications are greatly influenced by level of education, understanding of illness, understanding of treatment, familial support, past experiences, and, of course, one's own psychopathology.

The research on specific attitudes towards psychotropic medications in developing countries is limited, with most studies performed among different ethnic groups in high income countries. Comparing these groups to the indigenous counterparts in their countries of origin should be done with caution given that levels of education and environmental influences may vary. The acculturation process and effects of discrimination, along with socioeconomic disadvantages in this population, may have significant impact. However, these studies highlight the importance of managing expectations and learning about your population before treating blindly. One such study conducted in the US showed that Caucasians were more likely to take medication for depression compared to African-Americans and Hispanics, who preferred counseling and prayer as a means of treatment. This difference may be due to their other finding, that ethnic minorities were more likely to believe antidepressant medications were addictive (Givens et al. 2007). In another study, students in the UK were surveyed about their beliefs and experiences with medications. Those with Asian backgrounds indicated more negative views about medication than those who reported a European cultural background. And, similarly to the previously mentioned study, they were more likely to perceive medications as being harmful, possibly addictive substances that should be avoided (Horne et al. 2004). Other research studying psychotropic medication adherence in different ethnic populations showed lower rates of medication adherence in African-Americans and Hispanics compared to Caucasians (Diaz, Woods, & Rosenheck 2005).

Differences in pharmacokinetics across racial groups

The effect of a specific medication is determined by a multitude of factors. While pharmacokinetics (how the body utilizes, metabolizes, and eliminates a drug) are of great importance, the effects of diet, climate, and environmental exposure to other compounds all play a role. The placebo effect, which incidentally remains poorly understood and studied, demonstrates the hugely significant impact of the psyche in how our bodies will react to medications.

Differences in how the liver metabolizes a certain drug will determine blood levels and elimination. In particular, the role of specific enzymes (cytochrome P450) has been identified as a key player in this process. Many psychoactive medications are metabolized this way. Racial and thus genetic differences in how active these enzymes are consequently modify the amount of drug circulating within the body. Other effects include the rate of absorption through the gut and how quickly a drug is deactivated before it reaches the brain (DeVane 2009). Here we take a look at how the metabolism of some of the major psychotropic medication classes varies among ethnic groups.

- Antipsychotics. People of east-Asian descent have been shown to be more sensitive to antipsychotic medications such as haloperidol. They tend to show higher blood concentrations compared to Caucasians (Burroughs, Maxey, & Levy 2002; Wood & Zhou 1991). The practitioner treating this population should therefore use caution and not reflexively titrate these medications to doses normally used to treat Caucasians. There have not been significant differences in metabolism identified between people of African descent vs. Caucasians, though studies have shown that psychiatrists in the US tend to use higher doses of antipsychotics in African-American patients, possibly due to negative stereotyping (Strickland et al. 1991).
- Antidepressants. Most studies examining differences in metabolism have been conducted using tricyclic antidepressants. While these medications are no longer considered first-line treatment in developed countries, their use remains a pillar of treatment for depression in many developing countries. Similarly to antipsychotics, Asians (predominantly Chinese) have been shown to require lower doses of tricyclic antidepressants than Caucasians. Patients of African descent also appear to evidence higher blood concentrations than Caucasians despite taking

the same doses. Hispanics seem to require lower doses, though even at these lower doses they report a higher incidence of side effects (Burroughs et al. 2002; Wood & Zhou 1991).

- Benzodiazepines. There is only limited data available for this class of medications, but evidence suggests, once again, that Asians require lower doses of benzodiazepines. It is unclear whether this is due to differences in metabolism or average amount of body fat and volume of distribution (Burroughs et al. 2002; Wood & Zhou 1991).
- Lithium. Although there seems to be little difference in metabolism rates between ethnic groups, Asians are considered more sensitive to lithium. Consequently, they show the same improvement in symptoms at lower plasma levels compared to Caucasians (Lin, Poland, & Lesser 1986).

Practical considerations

The vignette described at the beginning of this chapter exemplifies an all-too-frequent occurrence in the developing world: medications that are needed cannot be obtained. The global mental health professional will be required to show flexibility and skill in utilizing the limited armamentarium of medications.

In the particular case described above, we have a patient who has been shown to respond to a particular antidepressant, venlafaxine. So far in our travels we have yet to encounter a developing country that stocks this particular medicine in their state formulary. We invite the reader to consider how they would manage this situation. Do you treat the patient with amitriptyline and hope for the best? Should you consider augmenting with other agents such as risperidone and/or lithium right away? If available, should ECT be considered? Can venlafaxine be obtained elsewhere?

In addition, we should also consider the implications of this general scenario: do you treat all depressed patients with amitriptyline, if that is the only drug readily available?

In our experience, one of the best tools to utilize when working in resource-scarce settings is knowledge. The following checklist will provide the global mental health professional with a guideline to being adequately equipped.

- ✓ Before traveling to your destination, ensure you have an accurate understanding of the social health care system and how the general population obtains medications.
- ✓ Learn what medications are generally available through the social health care system and at what cost.
- ✓ Ensure that you are well versed in prescribing the available medications, including off-label use.
- ✓ Learn what other medications are available in private pharmacies and what their cost is. It is important to understand how affordable these medications are to the general population.
- ✓ Try to gain an understanding of existing local prescribing practices, including traditional herbs/remedies/supplements. Familiarize yourself as much as possible with their efficacy.
- ✓ Learn what other treatment modalities, such as ECT, are available.

✓ Gain an understanding of the local burden of substance abuse and any available interventions.

✓ Consider the local population's attitude towards taking medication. For instance, would it be helpful to enlist the help of the family to ensure compliance, or would stigma towards pharmacotherapy only decrease compliance?

✓ Learn to 'think outside the box': if appropriate pharmacological treatment is not available, are there other interventions that could be beneficial/therapeutic? Explore support systems, vocational activities, enlisting non-mental-health providers, partnering with traditional healers, etc.

Perhaps one of the most important pharmacological considerations is to try to influence the availability of medications to the local population. This falls into the category of advocacy and should remain high on the global health practitioner's list of priorities.

References

Baldessarini, R. 2013, *Chemotherapy in Psychiatry,* 3rd edn, Springer, New York.

Biederman, J. 2003, 'Pharmacotherapy for attention-deficit/hyperactivity disorder (ADHD) decreases the risk for substance abuse: findings from a longitudinal follow-up of youths with and without ADHD,' *Journal of Clinical Psychiatry,* vol. 64, pp. 3–8.

Bowden, C. 2009, 'Valproate' in A. Schatzberg & C. Nemeroff (eds.), *The American Psychiatric Publishing Textbook of Psychopharmacology,* 4th edn, American Psychiatric Publishing, Arlington, VA.

Burroughs, V.J., Maxey, R.W., & Levy, R.A. 2002, 'Racial and ethnic differences in response to medicines: towards individualized pharmaceutical treatment,' *Journal of the National Medical Association,* vol. 94, no. 10 Suppl, pp. 1–26.

Clayton, A. & Gillespie, E. 2009, 'Bupropion' in A. Schatzberg & C. Nemerof (eds.), *The American Psychiatric Publishing Textbook of Psychopharmacology,* 4th edn, American Psychiatric Publishing, Arlington, VA.

Creese, A., Gasman, N., Mariko, M., & World Health Organization 2004, *The World Medicines Situation,* World Health Organization, Geneva.

Degenhardt, L., Whiteford, H.A., Ferrari, A.J., Baxter, A.J., Charlson, F.J., Hall, W.D., et al. 2013, 'Global burden of disease attributable to illicit drug use and dependence: findings from the Global Burden of Disease Study 2010,' *The Lancet,* vol. 382, no. 9904, pp. 1564–1574.

DeVane, L. 2009, 'Principles of pharmacokinetics and pharmacodynamics' in A. Schatzberg & C. Nemerof (eds.), *The American Psychiatric Publishing Textbook of Psychopharmacology,* 4th edn, American Psychiatric Publishing, Arlington, VA.

Diaz, E., Woods, S.W., & Rosenheck, R.A. 2005, 'Effects of ethnicity on psychotropic medications adherence,' *Community Mental Health Journal,* vol. 41, no. 5, pp. 521–537.

Freeman, M., Wiegand, C., & Gelenberg, A. 2009, 'Lithium' in A. Schatzberg & C. Nemerof (eds.), *The American Psychiatric Publishing Textbook of Psychopharmacology,* 4th edn, American Psychiatric Publishing, Arlington, VA.

Givens, J.L., Houston, T.K., Van Voorhees, B.W., Ford, D.E., & Cooper, L.A. 2007, 'Ethnicity and preferences for depression treatment,' *General Hospital Psychiatry,* vol. 29, no. 3, pp. 182–191.

Goff, D. 2009, 'Risperidone and Paliperidone' in A. Schatzberg & C. Nemerof (eds.), *The American Psychiatric Publishing Textbook of Psychopharmacology,* 4th edn, American Psychiatric Publishing, Arlington, VA.

Horne, R., Graupner, L., Frost, S., Weinman, J., Wright, S.M., & Hankins, M. 2004, 'Medicine in a multi-cultural society: the effect of cultural background on beliefs about medications,' *Social Science & Medicine,* vol. 59, no. 6, pp. 1307–1313.

Kemp, D., Muzina, D., Gao, K., & Calabrese, J. 2009, 'Lamotrigine' in A. Schatzberg & C. Nemerof (eds.), *The American Psychiatric Publishing Textbook of Psychopharmacology,* 4th edn, American Psychiatric Publishing, Arlington, VA.

Krafts, K., Hempelmann, E., & Skórska-Stania, A. 2012, 'From methylene blue to chloroquine: a brief review of the development of an antimalarial therapy,' *Parasitology Research,* vol. 111, no. 1, pp. 1–6.

Lin, K., Poland, R.E., & Lesser, I.M. 1986, 'Ethnicity and psychopharmacology,' *Culture, Medicine and Psychiatry,* vol. 10, no. 2, pp. 151–165.

Marder, S. & Wirshing, D. 2009, 'Clozapine' in A. Schatzberg & C. Nemerof (eds.), *The American Psychiatric Publishing Textbook of Psychopharmacology,* 4th edn, American Psychiatric Publishing, Arlington, VA.

Nelson, C. 2009, 'Tricyclic and tetracyclic drugs' in A. Schatzberg & C. Nemerof (eds.), *The American Psychiatric Publishing Textbook of Psychopharmacology,* 4th edn, American Psychiatric Publishing, Arlington, VA.

Polanczyk, G., de Lima, M., Horta, B., Biederman, J., & Rohde, L. 2007, 'The worldwide prevalence of ADHD: a systematic review and metaregression analysis,' *American Journal of Psychiatry,* vol. 164, no. 6, pp. 942–948.

Quirke, V.M. 2001, 'History of penicillin,' *eLS,* DOI: 10.1038/npg.els.0003626.

Reich, M.R. 1987, 'Essential drugs: economics and politics in international health,' *Health Policy,* vol. 8, no. 1, pp. 39–57.

Resolution, W. 1975, '28.66,' *Official Records of the WHO,* no. 226, pp. 35–36.

Sacks, L.V. & Behrman, R.E. 2008, 'Developing new drugs for the treatment of drug-resistant tuberculosis: a regulatory perspective,' *Tuberculosis,* vol. 88, pp. S93–S100.

Schatzberg, A. 2009, 'Mirtazapine' in A. Schatzberg & C. Nemerof (eds.), *The American Psychiatric Publishing Textbook of Psychopharmacology,* 4th edn, American Psychiatric Publishing, Arlington, VA.

Schatzberg, A., Cole, J., & DeBattista, C. 2010, 'Pharmacotherapy for substance use disorders' in A. Schatzberg, J. Cole, & C. DeBattista (eds.), *Manual of Clinical Psychopharmacology,* 7th edn, American Psychiatric Publishing, Arlington, VA.

Shaw, M., Hodgkins, P., Caci, H., Young, S., Kahle, J., Woods, A.G., & Arnold, L.E. 2012, 'A systematic review and analysis of long-term outcomes in attention deficit hyperactivity disorder: effects of treatment and non-treatment,' *BMC Medicine,* vol. 10, no. 1, p. 99.

Sheehan, D. & Raj, A. 2009, 'Benzodiazepines' in A. Schatzberg & C. Nemerof (eds.), *The American Psychiatric Publishing Textbook of Psychopharmacology,* 4th edn, American Psychiatric Publishing, Arlington, VA.

Shen, W.W. 1999, 'A history of antipsychotic drug development,' *Comprehensive Psychiatry,* vol. 40, no. 6, pp. 407–414.

Shorter, E. 1997, *A History of Psychiatry: From the Era of the Asylum to the Age of Prozac,* John Wiley & Sons Inc., New York.

Stanilla, J. & Simpson, G. 2009, 'Drugs to treat extrapyramidal side effects' in A. Schatzberg & C. Nemerof (eds.), *The American Psychiatric Publishing Textbook of Psychopharmacology,* 4th edn, American Psychiatric Publishing, Arlington, VA.

Strickland, T.L., Ranganath, V., Lin, K., Poland, R.E., Mendoza, R., & Smith, M. 1991, 'Psychopharmacologic considerations in the treatment of Black American populations,' *Psychopharmacology Bulletin,* vol. 27, no. 4, pp.441–448.

Thase, M. & Sloan, D. 2009, 'Venlafaxine and Desvenlafaxine' in A. Schatzberg & C. Nemerof (eds.), *The American Psychiatric Publishing Textbook of Psychopharmacology,* 4th edn, American Psychiatric Publishing, Arlington, VA.

Thullier, J. 1999, *Ten Years that Changed the Face of Mental Illness,* Taylor & Francis, London.

Whiteford, H.A., Degenhardt, L., Rehm, J., Baxter, A.J., Ferrari, A.J., Erskine, H.E., et al. 2013, 'Global burden of disease attributable to mental and substance use disorders: findings from the Global Burden of Disease Study 2010,' *The Lancet,* vol. 382, no. 9904, pp. 1575–1586.

Wilens, T.E., Faraone, S.V., Biederman, J., & Gunawardene, S. 2003, 'Does stimulant therapy of attention-deficit/hyperactivity disorder beget later substance abuse? A meta-analytic review of the literature,' *Pediatrics,* vol. 111, no. 1, pp. 179–185.

Wood, A.J. & Zhou, H.H. 1991, 'Ethnic differences in drug disposition and responsiveness,' *Clinical Pharmacokinetics,* vol. 20, no. 5, pp. 350–373.

World Health Organization, 1977, *The Selection of Essential Drugs: Report of a WHO Expert Committee,* WHO, Geneva.

World Health Organization 2001, *How To Develop and Implement a National Drug Policy,* WHO, Geneva.

World Health Organization 2014, *WHO Expert Committees.* Available: www.who.int/selection_medicines/committees/en/ (accessed October 19, 2014).

Zahajszky, J., Rosenbaum, J., & Tollefson, G. 2009, 'Fluoxetine' in A. Schatzberg & C. Nemerof (eds.), *The American Psychiatric Publishing Textbook of Psychopharmacology,* 4th edn, American Psychiatric Publishing, Arlington, VA.

Chapter 6

Psychotherapy

Sam has not been taking his antidepressant, and has little reason to, as far as he is concerned. How would a pill bring back his wife and children? And how would a pill take away this feeling of loneliness, which renders him exhausted and barely able to work in the fields?

The woman selling fruit on the roadside is Rose, a bright and energetic mother of four, who lost her husband during the war. She grew up in a village, the oldest of seven, raised by her parents who were both kind and caring people. Her father was a primary school teacher and would not let any of his children remain illiterate or uneducated. Rose therefore moved to the city when she was a teenager in order to attend high school. After graduating she met her husband, a clerk in the Ministry of Health, and soon started having children. A dedicated mother and community member, she found herself struggling after her husband died and started selling fruit in order to make ends meet.

Let us imagine that a new mental health initiative, organized by the Ministry of Health, is training lay people to deliver care in the form of counseling. Rose's husband had many friends at the Ministry who to this day try to take care of her and the children. She is approached by one of them asking if she might be interested in becoming a lay counselor. Given her disposition, her natural ability to take care of people, and her literacy, he feels she would be perfect for the job.

In the developed world, psychotherapy is considered an alternative or complementary treatment to medications for illnesses such as depressive- and anxiety disorders (Cuijpers et al. 2013). Cognitive behavioral therapy (CBT) is even emerging as an additional tool in the treatment of schizophrenia and other psychotic illnesses (Zimmermann et al. 2005). Several psychotherapy modalities, such as CBT and interpersonal therapy (IPT), have solid data supporting their efficacy as standalone treatments, making them a viable option for patients averse to taking medications (Cuijpers et al. 2013). Research has shown that psychotherapy can have a direct effect on gene expression and can alter the strength of neuronal connections (Karlsson 2011). In the developing world, with an ever-present shortage of appropriate psychotropic medications, such alternatives may represent the *only* options at times. However, in most places of the world, trained psychotherapists are de facto non-existent. This is one of the main barriers to providing psychological interventions worldwide (Patel et al. 2011). The solution to this problem is exemplified by the idea of task shifting: training non-psychiatric health care professionals and lay people to effectively provide psychotherapy to groups or individuals. We will take a look at the role of research—the studies that have been conducted to date and the need for further work to help solidify the development and implementation of psychotherapy in the developing world. The other main barrier is the cultural acceptability and appropriateness of psychological treatments that were developed in different cultural and socioeconomic contexts. We will discuss cross-cultural considerations to implementing psychotherapy in the developing world and take a look at issues such as confidentiality and culture-related attitudes towards 'opening up.' Finally, we will provide a scenario of what a psychotherapist trained in the developing world might encounter during their endeavors to bring their expertise to underserved parts of the world.

Task shifting

The WHO has acknowledged the importance of psychological treatments and has included recommendations for the treatment of several psychiatric disorders in its mhGAP Intervention Guide (WHO 2010). The following treatments are acknowledged and recommended:

- Cognitive Behavioral Therapy (CBT): a treatment focusing on changing negative thinking and/or behavior. It is recommended for the treatment of depression, behavioral disorders, alcohol and drug use disorders, and psychosis.
- Interpersonal Therapy (IPT): a treatment for depression based on the idea that interpersonal problems can lead to a depressed mood.
- Behavioral Activation Therapy: a treatment focusing on activity scheduling to help patients engage in rewarding activities. Recommended for depression.
- Motivational Enhancement Therapy: a treatment for substance abuse disorders focusing on motivating the individual to change their behavior.
- Contingency Management Therapy: a treatment used to reward desired behaviors and extinguish negative behaviors. It is used in substance abuse disorders.
- Parent skills training: a technique used to teach parents how to actively manage children with behavioral or developmental problems as well as improve their relationship and communication with them.
- Problem Solving Therapy: a basic counseling therapy aimed at providing direct and practical support for the individual. It is considered helpful with nearly any psychiatric condition.
- Relaxation Training: involves several techniques used to help alleviate anxiety and stress. It can be utilized for a multitude of disorders.
- Social Skills Training: a technique using role-playing, encouragement, and positive reinforcement to help rebuild skills and cope in social situations. It is recommended for individuals with psychotic disorders or behavioral problems.

In Chapter 2 we discussed the (often times lacking) human resources that are required to provide adequate mental health care in the developing world. Psychiatrists are an all-too-rare resource in these settings and it therefore falls on other professionals and lay people to provide the bulk of psychiatric care worldwide. Given that prescribing and managing medications is a complex skill, one that should require a fair amount of medical knowledge, we cannot expect non-medical providers to fulfill this task. Psychological treatments, such as counseling or psychotherapy, on the other hand, can be fairly easily rendered by health care workers without a psychiatric background, and, as research has shown, can even be taught to lay-people. This concept, otherwise referred to as *task shifting,* has been explored and researched in several trials. Here we will take a look at three of those trials, conducted in Uganda, Pakistan, and India, which have successfully shown how individuals without prior mental health care training can provide psychological-based treatments.

Trials

Uganda

In 2002 Bolton and colleagues studied whether group interpersonal therapy could successfully be implemented by lay health workers to help villagers in rural Uganda suffering from depression (Bolton et al. 2003). The group of lay health workers consisted of men and women, most of them between the ages of 18–22 and all of them high-school completers. None of them had a background in health care and all were trained during a 10-day intensive residential 'boot camp' using traditional lectures, modeling, and role-playing. After their training was complete, the lay health workers conducted group IPT on a weekly basis for 16 sessions. Patients receiving this type of treatment showed a significant reduction in depression scores at the time of termination and at six months following termination.

Pakistan

Rahman and colleagues conducted a trial in rural Pakistan studying the impact of cognitive behavioral therapy on pregnant women with depression (Rahman et al. 2008). The therapeutic interventions were implemented by village-based female health workers (so-called 'Lady Health Workers'), who had received a two-day training course. These women had completed secondary school, and had initially trained to provide mainly preventive maternal and child health care, as well as education in their communities. While they were not considered lay-people, they had no background in mental health and their routine work was enhanced by teaching them cognitive and behavioral techniques. The study showed a significant reduction in depression scores in women seen by these specially trained health workers, compared to the regular Lady Health Workers.

India

In a large-scale study in Goa, India, Patel et al. provided enhanced psychiatric treatment to patients in public and private primary care clinics. The treatment was delivered in part by lay health counselors who had been trained for two months. This group of lay counselors consisted of women, most of them with college degrees, who had no background in health care. The counselors acted as case managers, providing psychoeducation as well as psychotherapy (IPT) in close collaboration with primary care physicians. The control group received care from primary physicians who had access to a psychiatric treatment manual. The results of this trial showed an improved outcome in the intervention arm in public clinics but no significant difference in private clinics (Patel et al. 2010).

All of the above trials have successfully shown that lay workers, some with and some without higher education, can be utilized to provide important care to the mentally ill. And given the scarcity of professionals and abundance of untrained and unemployed individuals in the developing world, investing time and money in training these individuals can have a profound impact on the treatment of millions of patients. It is therefore with great enthusiasm that we recommend the global mental health professional consider this strategy as a viable option for increasing access to care in their community.

Cross-cultural considerations

Psychotherapy has been defined as the 'interaction of one person with another (or with others) by verbal means for the alleviation of emotional distress or for change in behavioral dysfunction' (Wittkower & Warms 1974). While psychotherapy was formally conceptualized and first researched in the late 19th and early 20th century, the idea of receiving help by talking to a fellow human being is as old as humankind itself. Different societies and cultures have established their own concepts of how an individual can seek help and what to expect from others. The individual in need of help can seek out an elder, a healer, or a group (family or otherwise) and share, to varying degrees of intimacy and disclosure, the nature of his or her concerns. Given the multitude of cultures and schools of thought, it is not surprising that various types of psychotherapies have evolved over time. The psychiatrist Jerome Frank pointed out that despite their individual differences, psychotherapies worldwide share the following similarities (Frank 1972):

1   An intense, emotionally charged, confiding relationship with a helping person.
2   A rationale, or myth, which includes an explanation of the cause of the patient's distress and a method for relieving it.
3   Provision of new information concerning the nature and sources of the patient's problems and possible alternative ways of dealing with them.
4   Strengthening the patient's expectations of help through the personal qualities of the therapist, enhanced by their status in society and the setting in which they work.
5   Provision of success experiences which further heighten the patient's hopes and also enhance their sense of mastery, interpersonal competence, or capability.

While these similarities highlight the universality of the human condition, effective psychotherapy also requires an understanding of the patient's culture, beliefs, and attitudes towards 'opening up.' A therapist from the United States should not expect to be able to successfully treat a patient from Uganda without first understanding the cultural context of their encounter. The following is a selection of factors that will influence an individual's view of the therapeutic process.

1   Family. In many societies it is the family's duty and responsibility to take care of its members. Opening up to strangers outside of the family may therefore be considered taboo or even shameful (Saveripillai & Schuetz-Mueller 2014; Soliman 1991). In addition, an individual may feel that his or her family will have access to the content of a therapeutic session.

2   Government. Societies that are governed through authoritarian power structures give little to no importance to the idea of freedom of choice. Individuals in these countries may have a very different sense of safety and confidentiality with their therapist or counselor.

3   Conceptualization of cause of distress. A patient who believes his or her distress is caused by a deity or evil spirit will have different expectations from a helping practitioner than a patient who believes their distress originates from an interpersonal problem.

4   Language. A society's understanding of mental illness is reflected in the local language. A therapist using local language and concepts will have a higher likelihood of reaching a patient. Using language that has not been adapted to the local culture will lead to confusion and alienation of the patient. For instance, many cultures lack a direct translation of the word *depression*, and instead describe syndromes with similar symptomatology. In Uganda two syndromes, *y'okwetchawa* and *okwekubaziga* were identified that met DSM-IV criteria of depression, but also contained other locally reported symptoms such as 'hating the world' and being unappreciative of assistance (Verdeli et al. 2003).

5   Attitude towards authority figures. Given that formal therapists or counselors have a high likelihood of being perceived as authority figures, the patient's attitude towards these figures will be reflected in the treatment. While this may vary highly between individuals, the therapist should be aware of the cultural perceptions of authority figures. For instance, Turkish psychotherapists conducting psychodynamic psychotherapy were reported to take a more action-oriented approach compared to US therapists given the more passive-dependent, expectant attitude towards clinicians (Ozturk & Volkan 1971).

In addition to these general factors that play a role in the therapeutic process, we should also consider the specific scenario of a global mental health practitioner providing psychotherapy as an outsider. The interplay between the practitioner's cultural, ethnic, educational, and geographic background with the patient's background will likely dictate some aspects of the therapeutic relationship. For instance, a patient may feel particularly eager to engage with a practitioner from afar if they feel this outsider will have superior qualifications and skills to provide help. In contrast, a patient from a country with a history of colonization sitting opposite a practitioner from the former colonial power may experience a sense of mistrust.

Practical guidelines

In our efforts to improve access to psychiatric care in underserved countries, we have consistently encountered a lack of available therapists and counselors to provide psychological treatments. Ironically, we encountered these very same challenges at home in New York, where, faced with a lack of resources for uninsured patients, we established a psychotherapy group for uninsured Spanish-speaking patients of East Harlem (Arroyo, Steinberg, & Katz 2012). The global mental health professional seeking to enhance a community's access to psychotherapy faces a challenging but achievable task. The following guidelines should provide a springboard for developing a counseling program.

1   Laying the groundwork: the first step consists of obtaining information surrounding the local culture of counseling/psychotherapy.

    a   Obtain an overview of the availability of human resources (if any) to provide formal counseling or psychotherapy.

        i   Are there mental health professionals available?
        ii   Are there other types of counselors available, such as HIV counselors, maternity health workers etc.?
        iii   What level of training and skillsets do existing counselors have?
        iv   What interventions do individuals expect to receive from these providers and are these acceptable to them?
        v   What role does confidentiality play in counseling?
        vi   What is the process wherein an individual seeks care with these professionals?
        vii   How are these providers funded?
        viii   Is their role captured in a local Mental Health Policy document?

    b   Learn about existing informal counseling resources and customs.

        i   What role do traditional healers/family/elders play in providing advice/counseling?
        ii   What interventions do individuals expect and receive from these informal resources?
        iii   What is the process wherein an individual seeks care with these informal resources?

    c   Understand the factors that determine whether an individual will seek formal or informal care.
    d   Understand the predominant conceptualization of common psychiatric conditions and their etiology.

        i   Learn what language is used to describe these conditions.
        ii   Learn about the local manifestation and symptomatology of common psychiatric conditions.

2   Preparing for action. Once you have an understanding of the availability of resources and the local customs you can move towards designing a program. Keep in mind that early interventions should be implemented on a small scale. This will enable you to easily fine tune your interventions and, once successful, provide justification to scale up.

    a   Identify stakeholders. Enhancing the delivery of psychotherapeutic interventions will require buy-in from local stakeholders, as they hold the key to financial assistance and the allocation of human resources. These stakeholders may be government officials, local medical directors, and mental health practitioners, among others. See Chapter 15 for further information.

b   Upgrading. If psychiatrically trained health workers are available (mental health nurses, psychiatric nurse practitioners, psychologists, psychiatrists), consider training them to enhance their skills to include psychotherapy. For example, existing psychiatric nurse practitioners at one of our collaborative sites were trained to provide CBT, a skill they had been lacking.

c   Task shifting. If non-psychiatric health workers are available, determine whether they can be utilized for mental health care or whether they can include mental health care in their work. For example, we encountered under-utilized HIV counselors in one of our collaborative sites, who were then trained in CBT to provide treatment for depression. As described in the study conducted in Pakistan (Rahman et al. 2008), maternity health workers were trained to include psychological interventions for pregnant women with depression.

d   Lay workers. Consider utilizing non-health care workers to provide psychological interventions. Keep in mind that these can be very cost effective and can provide care in groups to maximize the impact of their interventions.

e   Consider partnering and collaborating with existing traditional healers. If amenable, they could be trained to provide adapted psychological treatment. If not amenable, consider partnering with them to provide you with a referral base.

f   Consider partnering with an NGO invested in your cause. It may provide you with additional assistance as well as much-needed financial aid. In addition, many NGOs and/or global health programs are interested in conducting implementation research, which can open the door to further financial aid as well as provide you with evidence-based justifications for growing your program.

3   Training. Once you have devised an appropriate action plan for improving access to psychotherapy in your community you are ready to start training your future counselors/therapists.

a   Determine most appropriate framework. Whether individual CBT or group IPT, you should identify a therapy modality that has evidence-base for your purposes. As described above, CBT has been utilized to treat depression and can be taught fairly easily to lay workers, given its manualized approach. In order to maximize access to care, consider training in group therapy. As has been shown, group IPT has been effectively implemented to treat depression (Bolton et al. 2003; Verdeli et al. 2003).

b   Adapt your training to reflect local customs/beliefs/attitudes. With the knowledge you acquired during your initial phase of preparation, adapt treatment manuals to fit with local customs/beliefs and attitudes. Doing so in collaboration with local stakeholders and leaders will maximize your success. Reviewing existing literature on the topic may save you valuable time, given that a particular adaptation suiting your needs has already been developed.

c   Identify trainers. These may be local mental health practitioners, visiting physicians, collaborators from NGOs or global mental health programs.

d   Devise a training program. Develop a reasonable and affordable training program for the future mental health counselors while considering factors such as availability of trainers, costs, supplies, etc. Collaborating with stake-holders, NGOs, and global health programs is vital to this process.

e   Training. Train your future mental health counselors/therapists. Do so using different didactic approaches, such as lectures, discussions, experiential learning, role-playing, workbooks, case presentations, and videos. Ensure a solid understanding of the material has been achieved and ask for feedback on the training in order to further refine the process down the line. Also try to arrange for refresher courses after several months to further solidify the knowledge.

f   Supervision. Ensure that you are arranging for supervision once training is complete.

4   Implementation. This phase is where the actual clinical care is provided. Mental health counselors/therapists can now be deployed to do clinical work.

a   Provide adequate supervision. Especially early on, counselors will need guidance. Supervision can be done individually or in a group. If you have enlisted the help of remote experts, consider the utility of teleconferencing technology.

b   Ensure sustainability. In order to launch and maintain a successful program, you will need to prove its usefulness. Mental health counselors should keep track of their caseload and be able to create reports on productivity which can be utilized to justify ongoing support or scaling up of the program.

Returning to our vignette above, we can imagine a scenario in which both Rose's and Sam's life might change dramatically with the introduction of a task shifting initiative. When Sam returns to his doctor's office, with ongoing complaints of fatigue and depression, he tells his doctor of his reluctance to take medication. He feels it cannot solve his problems and he cannot remember to take them every day. His doctor, having been made aware of the new availability of lay counselors, sends Sam to see Rose. And while Sam is initially reluctant to speak with a woman he does not know, he feels comfortable knowing that she grew up in a village located not far from his own and understands some of the hardships he is facing.

References

Arroyo, H., Steinberg, E., & Katz, C.L. 2012, '"El Grupo": bringing psychotherapy to an underserved population,' *Psychiatric Services,* vol. 63, no. 7, pp. 718–718.

Bolton, P., Bass, J., Neugebauer, R., Verdeli, H., Clougherty, K.F., Wickramaratne, P., et al. 2003, 'Group interpersonal psychotherapy for depression in rural Uganda: a randomized controlled trial,' *JAMA: The Journal of the American Medical Association,* vol. 289, no. 23, pp. 3117–3124.

Cuijpers, P., Sijbrandij, M., Koole, S.L., Andersson, G., Beekman, A.T., & Reynolds, C.F. 2013, 'The efficacy of psychotherapy and pharmacotherapy in treating depressive and anxiety disorders: a meta-analysis of direct comparisons,' *World Psychiatry,* vol. 12, no. 2, pp. 137–148.

Frank, J.D. 1972, 'Common features of psychotherapy,' *Australasian Psychiatry,* vol. 6, no. 1, pp. 34–40.

Karlsson, H. 2011, 'How psychotherapy changes the brain,' *Psychiatric Times,* vol. 28, no. 8, pp. 21–23.

Ozturk, O.M. & Volkan, V.D. 1971, 'The theory and practice of psychiatry in Turkey,' *American Journal of Psychotherapy,* vol. 25, no. 2, pp. 240–271.

Patel, V., Chowdhary, N., Rahman, A., & Verdeli, H. 2011, 'Improving access to psychological treatments: lessons from developing countries,' *Behaviour Research and Therapy,* vol. 49, no. 9, pp. 523–528.

Patel, V., Weiss, H.A., Chowdhary, N., Naik, S., Pednekar, S., Chatterjee, S., et al. 2010, 'Effectiveness of an intervention led by lay health counsellors for depressive and anxiety disorders in primary care in Goa, India (MANAS): a cluster randomised controlled trial,' *The Lancet,* vol. 376, no. 9758, pp. 2086–2095.

Rahman, A., Malik, A., Sikander, S., Roberts, C., & Creed, F. 2008, 'Cognitive behaviour therapy-based intervention by community health workers for mothers with depression and their infants in rural Pakistan: a cluster-randomised controlled trial,' *The Lancet,* vol. 372, no. 9642, pp. 902–909.

Saveripillai, E.R. & Schuetz-Mueller, J. 2014, 'Annai Illam: using lay counselors to serve the trauma-related mental health needs of remote Sri Lanka,' *Annals of Global Health,* vol. 80, no. 2, pp. 122–125.

Soliman, A.M. 1991, 'The role of counseling in developing countries,' *International Journal for the Advancement of Counselling,* vol. 14, no. 1, pp. 3–14.

Verdeli, H., Clougherty, K., Bolton, P., Speelman, L., Lincoln, N., Bass, J., et al. 2003, 'Adapting group interpersonal psychotherapy for a developing country: experience in rural Uganda,' *World Psychiatry: Official Journal of the World Psychiatric Association (WPA),* vol. 2, no. 2, pp. 114–120.

Wittkower, E. & Warms, H. 1974, 'Cultural aspects of psychotherapy,' *Psychotherapy and psychosomatics,* vol. 24, no. 4–6, pp. 303–310.

World Health Organization 2010, *mhGAP Intervention Guide for Mental, Neurological And Substance Use Disorders in Non-specialized Health Settings: Mental Health Gap Action Programme (mhGAP),* WHO, Geneva.

Zimmermann, G., Favrod, J., Trieu, V., & Pomini, V. 2005, 'The effect of cognitive behavioral treatment on the positive symptoms of schizophrenia spectrum disorders: a meta-analysis,' *Schizophrenia Research,* vol. 77, no. 1, pp. 1–9.

Chapter 7

Traditional medicine

Off to the upper right in the photo is an unremarkable second story apartment that serves as the home of one of the traditional healers/herbalists who dot the country. He is home today because it is an auspicious occasion. His usual schedule would have seen him out for the day working his primary job as a carpenter. He usually comes back at night to find people lining up outside of his door to see him. They arrive without appointments and get seen one by one in his living room until no one is left.

He comes from a long lineage of healers, and it makes him feel good to use his god-given gifts for the benefit of others. He makes some money from it but has never turned away anyone for lack of ability to pay. He also donates half of his earnings to his local temple, where he occasionally also fills in as a priest.

The healer sees people for almost any problem, including physical complaints like headache and abdominal pain, possession by spirits or demons, infertility, or curses. He especially detests getting involved when family members curse one another, but sees it as his duty. His technique primarily relies on herbs, supplemented by prayer and special implements such as sacred threads, palm leaves, and coconut shells. He often relies on the wind when it is around in abundance, which is exactly what he did when Sam stopped by one his way back from the hospital. The healer still cannot understand why the big doctors at the hospital do not seek his opinion out for themselves.

The Western global mental health professional seeks to share their expertise with places in need. Their travel is premised on bringing health care in low and middle income countries and other low resource settings closer to the standards of Western practice. As such, they tend to interact with the local health and, where available, mental health systems in the host countries. However, many, if not most, places in the world have a parallel system of care founded in traditional, or folk-based, approaches to healing. In this chapter we will describe the nature and scope of traditional medicine around the world. We will then review what we know about it in relation to mental health and spell out the practical implications for global mental health practice.

Traditional medicine

The World Health Organization (2000) defines *traditional medicine* as

[T]he sum total of the knowledge, skills, and practices based on the theories, beliefs, and experiences indigenous to different cultures, whether explicable or not, used in the maintenance of health as well as in the prevention, diagnosis, improvement or treatment of physical and mental illness.

Traditional medicine is often used interchangeably with the terms complementary and alternative medicine (CAM) (Bodeker et al. 2005a). Complementary medicine can be defined as medicine given as a complement to conventional therapies, while alternative medicines are those which are given in its place (Mamtani & Cimino 2002).

More recently, CAM has been defined as a 'broad domain of healing resources that encompasses all health systems, modalities, and practices and their accompanying theories and beliefs, other than those intrinsic to the politically dominant health system of a particular society or culture in a given historical period' (Zollman & Vickers 1999). Generally speaking, Western or modern medicine with the WHO as its standard bearer and global mental health as an offshoot is the politically dominant health system in the world. On the other hand, traditional medicine in the guise of our healer from the photo involves health practices indigenous to the cultures visited by global mental health practitioners. We will use the term traditional medicine in this chapter as we believe it has more global currency than CAM.

Traditional medicine can be divided into five broad areas of practice, as follows: (1) alternative medicine systems (i.e. Chinese medicine, acupuncture, Ayuverda); (2) mind-body interventions (i.e., meditation, hypnosis, prayer); (3) biologically based therapies (i.e., herbal medicines); (4) manipulative and body based therapies (i.e., chiropractic and massage); and (5) energy therapies (i.e., Reiki) (Mamtani & Cimino 2002).

Traditional healers would then be the broad name for any practitioner of any such traditional medical practices, but the WHO (2014) has described six different types of traditional healers:

- Healers such as traditional health practitioners and herbalists who elicit symptoms and then prescribe herbs, medicines, or other physical treatments in a doctor-like fashion. They are themselves often specifically referred to as 'traditional healers.'
- Faith healers seek divine guidance and then prescribe treatments accordingly. They may also make offerings to the gods.
- Shamans believe that sickness occurs when someone's soul wanders away and fails to return. They rely on a trance like ritual to retrieve it.
- 'Witch doctors' attribute illness to spirits that have been cast into an individual's body by an offended spirit seeking revenge or by way of black magic cast by another person. They rely on diverse magic and rituals to help the afflicted person.
- Fortune tellers prognosticate how long someone will be sick, often relying on a trance state to discern this.
- Healers, including traditional birth attendants, who specialize in massage.

Availability of traditional medicine

In many parts of the world, people have far more access to traditional healing than they do modern medical care. In Africa, as much as 80 percent of the population

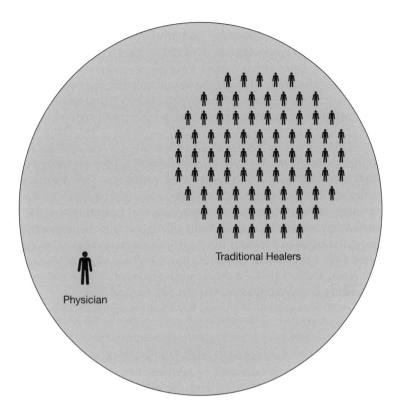

Figure 7.1 Ratio of traditional healers to Western medical practitioners in Sub-Saharan Africa per 40,000 population

Source: Truer 2007

depends upon traditional healers to meet their health care needs, while 70 percent do so in India (Bodeker et al. 2005a). In sub-Saharan Africa, estimates suggest that the ratio of healers to the population is 1:500 in comparison to 1:40,000 for Western medical providers (Figure 7.1). And, in South Africa alone in 1995, it was estimated that there were 200,000 practicing healers (Truter 2007). We have found that most traditional healers have more 'conventional' full time jobs and ply their healing craft part-time.

To the extent that data is available, rates of use of particular types of traditional medical practices vary quite widely around the world according to local customs and history. Chinese medicine and acupuncture are of course especially popular in China, as is Ayurveda in India. Chiropractic has a particular home in the US, while homeopathy is practiced extensively in Russia (Bodeker et al. 2005b). Different countries also have various levels of investment in and oversight of tradi-tional medicine. Some countries require that traditional healers undergo licensure, have educational institutions in traditional medicine, and have national expert com-mittees on the subject. Some even have lists of essential traditional medications (i.e., Pakistan).

Traditional practice and mental health

Frameworks for comparing Western/modern and traditional medical approaches to mental health diagnosis and treatment are depicted in Tables 7.1 and 7.2. Given the enormous variety in the types of traditional medical practices and practitioners, these are necessarily generalizations. In fact, the details are less important than the mindset. The two approaches are often very different in practice and spirit, but there is little to suggest that they are contradictory and ample room to embrace their complementarity.

Traditional healers often wind up addressing problems that we would call mental illness without calling it as such. And, as reflected in Table 7.1, they are likely to have very different beliefs about the nature and cause of the problems. This is reflected in a quote from a healer we met in Gujarat, India: 'If there are two people, and one guy has a feeling of revenge, the other person will have [acquire] mental illness. He may not be directly possessing him, but he may have the other guy drink something.' And, here are some characterizations of mental illness from healers in that same region: 'There are problems that affect mind and soul, but we don't identify as different problems. They are possessed by spirits.' Another healer intoned, 'There are problems which affect mind and soul, and the reason is nature (all nature).'

As for treating the problems related to mental health, here is one description from one of our trips to India:

> Do puja [prayer] and go to the mandir [Hindu temple]. If they follow the rules, they will get better. If the guy is possessed by demons, first they come to me, and I take them inside the temple, we pray, and the goddess comes into me. The

Table 7.1 Comparison of modern and traditional approaches to mental health diagnosis

MODERN medicine	vs.	TRADITIONAL medicine
Observation, interview, anamnesis, tests		Observation, interview, divination, mediumship
Manifest symptoms reflect latent intra-psychic factors		Manifest symptoms reflect latent supernatural factors

Source: Adapted from Okpaku 1998

Table 7.2 Comparison of modern and traditional approaches to mental health treatment

MODERN treatment	Vs.	TRADITIONAL treatment
Therapist-patient communication		Communication w/ supernatural agent
Verbal or behavioral		Ritualistic performance
Possible medication		Possible medication
Insight, transference, corrective behavior		Cleansing, exorcism, corrective behavior
Value = mastery		Value = harmony

Source: Adapted from Okpaku 1998

goddess [inside the healer] talks to the patient and makes the evil spirit inside the patient talk. She [goddess] asks 'what is the problem, why are you possessing?' The spirit says what they want and then we have to give that thing. Unless and until they get that thing, the spirit will live. The spirit says whatever it needs and we will get it (for example, something to eat) and the spirit will go away into the wind.

(Katz, unpublished data)

Another example incorporates dietary changes into the intervention:

When the patient comes here, first they make him pray to Devi Mata [Hindu goddess], then drink liquid which has lemon and sugar. He's supposed to drink it for 1 month, and for 1.5 months he's not supposed to take alcohol or non-veg [non-vegetarian], and supposed to pray to god. We pray for him on his behalf here in the temple.

(Katz, unpublished data)

Research on the traditional medicine modalities in the developed world has lent some support for its practice. For example, studies support the benefits of exercise and yoga, but not tai chi, meditation, or qigong, as alternative treatments for anxiety and depression (Saeed, Antonacci, & Bloch 2010). Herbal remedies appear to be effective and to have a highly desirable side-effect profile in late life depression (Nyer et al. 2013). Preliminary evidence suggests that yoga, meditation, exercise, massage, tai chi, spiritual therapy, and music therapy are also effective (Nyer et al. 2013). Emerging evidence supports the use of acupuncture for clinical depression and anxiety, whereas there is conflicting evidence for its use in substance use disorders and no data regarding schizophrenia (Samuels et al. 2008).

Still, traditional medicine is saddled with a dearth of data to support its practice. One review has found an overall lack of high quality or conclusive findings regarding traditional medicine and depression (Thachil, Mohan, & Bhugra 2007). Authoritative reviews have also found inadequate data on which to draw conclusions for or against traditional medicine in the following: exercise for childhood anxiety and depression (Larun et al. 2006); meditation for ADHD (Krisanaprakornkit et al. 2010); and, despite its popularity, meditation for anxiety (Krisanaprakornkit et al. 2006).

Studies on traditional medicine and mental health in the developing world tend to focus on the role and impact of traditional healers rather than specific remedies. In Pakistan, shamans serve as de facto psychotherapists, thereby compensating for the dearth of mental health professionals in that country (Gadit 2003). Among South Africans with a psychiatric disorder in a nationally representative sample, 29 percent reported seeking out a Western health professional and 20 percent, who were more likely to be black, unemployed, and less educated, saw a traditional healer. Investigators concluded that traditional healers provided a substantial portion of the mental health care in South Africa (Sorsdahl et al. 2009).

There is a considerable preponderance of studies on healing and mental health from India. A fascinating year-long study of a 10,000 member village in West India found that villagers often saw both traditional healers and physicians at the same time for a given mental health complaint and frequented many healers; all socioeconomic classes frequented healers; healers readily referred cases to physicians; and healers and physicians were in frequent agreement on the nature of their patients' problems (Kapur 1979). Indians often frequent 'healing temples' representing an array of religions to reside and recuperate from mental health conditions. In one naturalistic study, the majority of the 31 visitors were found to have schizophrenia and only one of them had ever seen a medical professional. They stayed for an average for six weeks, typically accompanied by family members. A significant reduction in psychopathology scores was noted across the visit, and, in the absence of any specific healing rituals, it was concluded that the non-threatening, supportive environment may have had a salutary effect (Raguram et al. 2002). A different study of patients of traditional and faith healers in South India found that the most common presenting problems were in the anxiety-depression spectrum (Shankar, Saravanan, & Jacob 2006).

Conclusions

It is our recommendation that you work with healers whenever possible. The reasons for doing so are at least clinical, organizational, and political in nature. First, consider them potential recruits in re-creating the multi-disciplinary approach to mental health care with which most Western mental health practitioners are familiar, even if with a very different kind of cross-cultural make-up. Second, traditional healers constitute the backbone of health care delivery in much of the world. Partnering with them would be akin to providing collaborative care with a primary care physician in America or elsewhere. Third, traditional healers have great influence and can serve as your liaisons to the local community.

Here is a guide for working with healers (WHO 2014):

✓ Familiarize yourself with the nature and extent of traditional medicine practice in your host country before going by consulting the WHO *Global Atlas of Traditional, Complementary, and Alternative Medicine* (text and map volumes) (Bodeket et al. 2005a, 2005b).
✓ For mental health clinicians, if you do not usually incorporate traditional medicine into your practice, consider consulting a comprehensive, if Western-oriented, book on the topic, *How to Use Herbs, Nutrients, & Yoga in Mental Health Care* (Brown, Gerbarg, & Muskin 2009).
✓ Communicate with your hosts about your intention to cooperate with local healers in order to seek out their help with identifying them. In our experience, healers are best found by word of mouth.
✓ Anticipate that your local medical colleagues may themselves treat local healers with suspicion and even derision.
✓ Show respect for the healers, if for no other reason than that they usually garner respect from their communities.
✓ Be humble about the capacities of Western medicine.
✓ Do not challenge healers, instead adopting a stance of collegial curiosity. What can you learn from them?
✓ Work with different healers, as there is often great variation in practice even within a given community.
✓ Rely on the community members to help identify trusted healers.

Remember that Sam stopped to see the healer even after making the long trip to the hospital and having the seeming good fortune to receive specialized Western psychiatric ministrations. In total, we therefore suggest you live by this 'golden rule'—the way to incorporate traditional healers into your global mental health work is to remember that in their country and in their community, they are the ones incorporating you.

References

Bodeker, G., Ong, C.K., Grundy, C., Burford, G., & Shein, K. 2005a, *WHO Global Atlas of Traditional, Complementary, and Alternative Medicine, Text Volume*, World Health Organization, Kobe, Japan.

Bodeker, G., Ong, C.K., Grundy, C., Burford, G., & Shein, K. 2005b, *WHO Global Atlas of Traditional, Complementary, and Alternative Medicine, Map Volume*, World Health Organization, Kobe, Japan.

Brown, R.R., Gerbarg, P.L., & Muskin, P.R. 2009, *How to Use Herbs, Nutrients, & Yoga in Mental Health Care*, W.W. Norton and Company, New York.

Gadit, A.A. 2003, 'Health services delivery by shamans: a local experience in Pakistan,' *International Journal of Mental Health*, vol. 32, no. 2, pp. 63–83.

Kapur, R. 1979, 'The role of traditional healers in mental health care in rural India,' *Social Science & Medicine. Part B: Medical Anthropology*, vol. 13, no. 1, pp. 27–31.

Krisanaprakornkit, T., Krisanaprakornkit, W., Piyavhatkul, N., & Laopaiboon, M. 2006, 'Meditation therapy for anxiety disorders,' *The Cochrane Database of Systematic Reviews*, vol. 1, no. 1, p. CD004998.

Krisanaprakornkit, T., Ngamjarus, C., Witoonchart, C., & Piyavhatkul, N. 2010, 'Meditation therapies for attention-deficit/hyperactivity disorder (ADHD),' *The Cochrane Database of Systematic Reviews*, vol. 6, no. 6, p. CD006507.

Larun, L., Nordheim, L.V., Ekeland, E., Hagen, K.B., & Heian, F. 2006, 'Exercise in prevention and treatment of anxiety and depression among children and young people,' *The Cochrane Database of Systematic Reviews*, vol. 3, no. 3, p. CD004691.

Mamtani, R. & Cimino, A. 2002, 'A primer of complementary and alternative medicine and its relevance in the treatment of mental health problems,' *Psychiatric Quarterly*, vol. 73, no. 4, pp. 367–381.

Nyer, M., Doorley, J., Durham, K., Yeung, A.S., Freeman, M.P., & Mischoulon, D. 2013, 'What is the role of alternative treatments in late-life depression?,' *The Psychiatric Clinics of North America*, vol. 36, no. 4, pp. 577–596.

Okpaku, S.O. (ed.) 1998, *Clinical Methods in Transcultural Psychiatry*, American Psychiatric Press, Washington, D.C., p. 96, Table 5.1.

Raguram, R., Venkateswaran, A., Ramakrishna, J., & Weiss, M.G. 2002, 'Traditional community resources for mental health: a report of temple healing from India,' *BMJ: British Medical Journal*, vol. 325, no. 7354, p. 38.

Saeed, S.A., Antonacci, D.J., & Bloch, R.M. 2010, 'Exercise, yoga, and meditation for depressive and anxiety disorders,' *American Family Physician*, vol. 81, no. 8, pp. 981–986.

Samuels, N., Gropp, C., Singer, S.R., & Oberbaum, M. 2008, 'Acupuncture for psychiatric illness: a literature review,' *Behavioral Medicine*, vol. 34, no. 2, pp. 55–64.

Shankar, B.R., Saravanan, B., & Jacob, K. 2006, 'Explanatory models of common mental disorders among traditional healers and their patients in rural south India,' *International Journal of Social Psychiatry*, vol. 52, no. 3, pp. 221–233.

Sorsdahl, K., Stein, D.J., Grimsrud, A., Seedat, S., Flisher, A.J., Williams, D.R., & Myer, L. 2009, 'Traditional healers in the treatment of common mental disorders in South Africa,' *The Journal of Nervous and Mental Disease*, vol. 197, no. 6, pp. 434–441.

Thachil, A.F., Mohan, R., & Bhugra, D. 2007, 'The evidence base of complementary and alternative therapies in depression,' *Journal of Affective Disorders*, vol. 97, no. 1–3, pp. 23–35.

Truter, I. 2007, 'African traditional healers: cultural and religious beliefs intertwined in a holistic way,' *SA Pharmaceutical Journal*, vol. 74, no. 8, pp. 56–60.

World Health Organization 2000, *General Guidelines for Methodologies on Research and Evaluation of Traditional Medicine*, World Health Organization, Geneva.

World Health Organization 2014, *Traditional Medicine and Traditional Healers*. Available: www.who.int/mental_health/resources/en/MNH%20of%20refugees_unit6_7pdf.pdf (accessed January 22, 2014).

Zollman, C. & Vickers, A. 1999, 'What is complementary medicine?,' *BMJ (Clinical research edn)*, vol. 319, no. 7211, pp. 693–696.

Part 3

Unique practice populations

Chapter 8

Children and adolescents

Linda Chokroverty, MD, FAAP

While walking wearily about the streets in the post-war capital, Sam notes an eerie absence of children at play, though an occasional boy is seen here and there. An older school aged boy is clearly visible in the foreground, sitting next to his mother the local produce vendor, and another younger boy with his schoolbag is looking on at some adults at what could be the counting of a ballot box. A boy upstairs with the herbalist could be a teenager, and in the distance, a shadowy figure of yet another boy lurks by a car . . . and finally, a brightly colored bundle on a mother's back might contain a baby. The fracture of family and normal childhood is palpable in the scene of boys and an infant, largely in isolation from their usual activity and social context, metaphorical for the fracture and sense of displacement and disorder felt by the community post conflict.

The concept of childhood invokes many attitudes and assumptions on the part of adults across historical, cultural, and professional contexts. The proverbs 'Children should be seen and not heard' (Aristophanes 423BC) and 'Spare the rod, spoil the child' (Samuel Butler, 17th century poet), connote historical opinion on the place of children and how they should be managed. Many of these attitudes assume a 'second class' role to children in the larger context of society. The expected role is generally one of passivity, never the center of attention from either a political or policy stand-point; one that serves as extensions of adults or families rather than as individuals; and generally one as objects for child-minding and 'mouths to feed,' rather than as those with their own unique character and needs that differ greatly from that of adults. The field of child and adolescent mental health is a vast one, but this chapter endeavors to provide an overview of key issues in the field relevant to global mental health practice, including mental health issues of children as individuals and as part of a larger social ecology; the mental health challenges faced by some children using a developmental perspective; some of the more common mental disorders encountered among children; and, finally, evidence informed treatment strategies in settings that may be resource poor.

Background

A child is broadly defined as 'a person under the age of 18' by the United Nations (Article 1, Convention of the Rights of the Child; UNICEF 2014).[1] A variety of international and local laws further define the minimum age at which the end of mandatory education, marriage, conscription, citizenship, employability, and criminality can occur. Culture and circumstances cause wide variation in interpretation of the boundaries of childhood, and despite the existence of many laws, violations occur often and regularly in much of the world that rob children of their childhood, forcing them to assume adulthood before they may be ready. Situations of poverty and economic hardship, war and other experiences of extreme violence and loss, local customs around early marriage, forced employment, and limits on educational opportunity all impact upon a community's interpretation of childhood.

Lower priority of children's needs compared to adults and fluid definitions of childhood do not imply, however, that progress has not been made in advocating for children's needs on a global scale. The World Health Organization and the United Nations for example have made considerable progress in improving the general health of children worldwide in the areas of infant mortality, nutrition, and disease prevention. To a lesser extent, progress in human rights and political advocacy of children have also been made. What lags far behind these advancements however, are child mental health awareness and efforts to foster good emotional development for children. As noted in Chapter 1, the importance of children as needing special attention for mental health disorder prevention and care has been identified by specialists and policymakers, but child mental health continues to receive less attention than adult mental health in middle and low income countries/low-resource settings (Collins et al. 2011; Morris et al. 2011).

Using our illustration of Sam and his community, let's take a look at the children and how they are depicted in the painting as a metaphor for both the seen and the unseen. What mental health questions might come to mind with these youngsters?

Let's look at the first boy reading the newspaper. One could argue that he is a bit odd, sitting with his mother and feet in the vegetable bin, whereas he might have been playing football with his peers in a nearby field if he were like other children. Perhaps he is on the autistic spectrum, classically known as 'savant,' advanced in a restricted way and yet immature, in need of his mother's supervision despite his older age and unable to engage his contemporaries. Now the other school aged boy facing away with his rucksack attending to the adults with the ballot box—why is he alone? One wonders where his classmates are as a child his age highly values peer friendships especially of the same gender. Perhaps this boy had been sent to the marketplace by his family to buy provisions but in typical child-like way becomes distracted by other developments in the area. Maybe he has a healthy interest in the rebuilding efforts of the community by way of election process and democracy.

Let's move up to the herbalist's office upstairs. That teenager there might be seeking remedy for drug addiction or anxiety brought on during and since his experience of having been abducted and released by a local gang where he was forced to participate in armed conflict against his own community.

What about the little baby on the mother's back—does her mother spend time interacting with and nurturing her at home? Maybe her mother can provide the attention and care that the baby needs. But if her mother were walking around in a 'daze' because her husband was killed during combat, the baby is just carried around all the time, otherwise neglected—yet another casualty of war.

Let us consider further what is missing and thereby truly unseen in this picture. Where are the younger children—the toddlers and preschool aged children? Perhaps they are being cared for at home with mothers who could not go into town. A more grim possibility is that a large portion of the younger children and their mothers have been wiped out in a cholera outbreak or detained in refugee camps, leaving returning husbands and fathers without families. Another scenario puts the infants and preschoolers out of the picture because they are orphans being looked after in a large home for displaced children whose parents were killed in the war. Where are the girls in this scene? Chances are they remain at home providing domestic work for the family instead of attending school or being out in the community. Could they have been marginalized from society for having been sexually abused, or conversely, could they be afraid to be out in public for fear of further harm and exploitation or simply shame? These questions and speculations raised by the illustration should heighten the mental health caregiver's attention to issues at the level of community, family, and individual, all of which impact upon the emotional development and wellbeing of children.

A framework of issues related to children's mental health

The authors suggest the following framework to conceptualize the types of variables that impact child mental health. Situational variables that impact the mental health of children occur at the three levels, as shown in Figure 8.1, namely, community, family, and individual (see Table 8.1). *Six major community level issues* can be identified as variables affecting child mental health, as follows: the presence of *war and terrorism* with an associated culture of violence, danger, corruption, crime, and unpredictability; severe *poverty* and limited economic opportunity (Albee 1986), related to or independent of the first variable of war/terrorism; the occurrence of *natural and other disaster* with associated destruction and disruption (Laor & Wilmer 2007), related to or independent of poverty, war/terrorism; *infectious disease* and problems with health care access (Prince et al. 2007), related to or independent of poverty, war, and disaster;

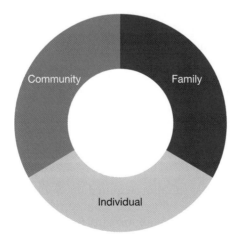

Figure 8.1 The three levels of impact on child mental health

Table 8.1 Dimensions of community, family, and the individual that affect children's mental health

Community	Family	Individual
War and terrorism	Loss of parent(s)	Congenital/developmental delays
Extreme poverty	Separation of family	Traumatic exposure
Natural and other disaster	Caregiver mental illness	Nutritional status
Access to health care	Financial hardship	Prolonged separation from
Educational opportunity		caregivers
Other community		Drug and alcohol use
resources		

educational opportunity (Patel & Kleinman 2003), related to or independent of poverty, war, and disaster; and, finally, the availability of *community resources* such as recreational institutions or facilities (libraries, playgrounds, and parks), cultural institutions, social organizations, places of worship, native healers, a functioning government and system of law enforcement, related to or independent of poverty, war, disaster. The last item of community resources facilitates social relationships among and within the community, a notion known as social capital, which has been tied to the wellbeing of children (Putnam et al. 2004; Morrow 2004).

The authors suggest *four important family variables* to the reader that impact upon child mental health. *First,* the violent and unexpected *loss of a parent*/primary caregiver can have devastating and enduring effects on a child's future development (Bowlby 1980). *Second, family economic hardship,* that results in inadequate nutrition, non-potable drinking water, and/or crowded living conditions can create physical as well as psychosocial stress for children, prenatally as well as postnatally (Albee 1986). *Third, parental reaction to stress* is an important determinant of a child's ability to cope with the same stressors. Maladaptive responses to stress such as parental depression, anxiety/post-traumatic stress symptoms, alcohol and drug abuse, aggression in the form of domestic violence have been shown to have highly negative effects on child mental health (Prince et al. 2007). The wellbeing of the parent is important to a child's health, as many cases have been seen where a baby does not gain weight and grow properly because the adult taking care of the baby is doing poorly and neglecting the needs of the infant by feeding him or her too little, or failing to provide the love and care required (McLean & Price 2011). *Fourth, separation from, dislocation, and/or displacement* of the family unit are associated with negative mental health effects (Fazel & Stein 2002), whereas correction of this variable through reunification and resettlement is associated with positive mental health effects on children (Betancourt 2010).

Five individual level variables impact child mental health using the authors' suggested framework. *First,* congenital or acquired *developmental delays/abnormalities* have an effect on emotional development. Congenital and acquired developmental abnormalities include chromosomal abnormalities, prenatal and postnatal exposures to toxins (e.g., heavy metals, drugs, or alcohol), infections, head trauma, or nutritional deficiencies, all of which can cause developmental impairments and in some cases, intellectual disability (formerly known as 'mental retardation') in children (Shapiro & Batshaw 2011; Feigelman 2011a; American Psychiatric Association, 2013). Walker et al. (2007) identified a number of modifiable biological and psycho-social risk factors that are linked with compromised development in children under 5. Of these, the ones that need urgent attention are growth stunting, inadequate cognitive stimulation, iodine deficiency, and iron deficiency anemia. Additional risk factors are identified in the review that also warrant attention including malaria, intrauterine growth restriction, maternal depression, exposure to violence, and exposure to heavy metals (Walker et al. 2007). For example, prenatal deficiency of the nutrient iodine leads to congenital hypothyroidism in the unborn infant and subsequent poor brain development including impaired intellectual development and cerebral palsy; as such iodine deficiency is noted to be the most common preventable cause of mental retardation (as noted, now known as intellectual disability) (Pharaoh & Connolly 1995; Walker et al. 2007). The impact of intellectual disability can be significant for the child and family. Severe intellectual disability can result in behavioral disturbances, and children of all degrees of intellectual disability are at risk for maltreatment by adults and other children who don't recognize their 'special needs' (Sullivan & Knutsen 2000). In the period of birth to age 5, brain infections (meningitis, encephalitis) can have dire neurologic and cognitive effects on future brain development (Prober & Dyner 2011). Malaria is an especially serious problem worldwide—in 2012 over 207 million cases were diagnosed, with children under 5 being the most at risk due to limited immunity (CDC 2014b). The population under 5, of course, is the most vulnerable from a developmental standpoint as well, and the effect of malarial infection upon the brain can be profound. Cognitive deficits may occur as a result of malarial infection not only for the most severe cases but also the less severe (Kihara et al. 2006). Autism Spectrum Disorder, commonly known as autism, is an under-recognized phenomenon that has serious future implications for a child's social and emotional health (American Psychiatric Association, 2013; Minshew & Payton 1988).

The *second* individual level variable in child mental health is *traumatic exposure*. These include life-threatening events, witnessed death or serious injury of close family members, severe physical injury, physical and sexual abuse. The likelihood of experiencing persistent post-traumatic stress symptoms (in the general categories of hyper-arousal, re-experiencing, and numbness) increases with a higher dose as well as cumulative amount of traumatic exposures (Stoddard 2014). In addition to Post-Traumatic Stress Disorder (PTSD), guilt, depression, suicidality, and externalizing behaviors have also been noted in child trauma survivors. The example of the child soldier presents a more recently recognized and special mental health challenge, as these children frequently experience a problem known as complex PTSD. This disorder (discussed again later) includes problems in affect regulation, memory and attention, self-perception, interpersonal relations, somatization, and systems of meaning (Herman, 1992). The *third individual variable* suggested by the authors affecting child mental health is receipt of *nourishment and nurturance*. This variable can include sufficient nutrition, immunization against disease/maintenance of health, educational enrichment and stimulation, supervision, protection from harm, and parental availability/engagement (Masten et al. 1990). In the first few years of life, lack of essential nutrients such as iron and fatty acids can cause inadequate myelination and other aspects of brain development that can in turn negatively impact the timely achievement of developmental milestones (Prado & Dewey 2014). These milestones are markers of normal motor, speech, cognitive, and emotional development, delays in which can have negative effects on child mental health (Emerson & Einfield 2010). The absence of nourishment and nurturance is a major cause of psychosocial failure to thrive seen most dramatically during infancy, but also over various periods of critical growth and development during childhood and adolescence (Wachs et al. 2014). The *fourth variable* is *prolonged separation* from parents and/or primary caregivers. A consistent and stable relationship with a mother or primary caregiver if the mother is not available is highly important to the infant and young child's development. This relationship of a mother–child bond helps the infant and young child practice interacting with another person, helps the child feel safe and cared for, and prepares the child for future relationships with other children and adults. Attachment problems are often seen with infants and very young children experiencing prolonged separation, highlighted especially among children in large, custodial care arrangements such as orphanages (discussed again later), but mitigated in cases of prompt surrogate caregiving and return of routine during the period of separation from parents (Kellmer Pringle & Bossio 1960). The *fifth variable* is childhood *drug and alcohol abuse*, which frequently relates to the other variables of traumatic exposure, failed nourishment in cases of poor supervision and neglect, and prolonged separation from caregivers (Saunders & Adams 2014).

Identification and assessment of mental disorders in children using a developmental approach

Also prompted by the scene in the book's overarching illustration are the importance of age specific developmental concerns in children and the challenge of achieving important developmental tasks as individuals within the general context and ecology of the child's life. One of the biggest challenges in working with children is that they present with distress and disability in a different way than do adults (Esposito et al. 2011). As a result, there is a greater need to do detective work on the part of the health care worker. The process of normal child development itself accounts for much of this challenge—children are continuously evolving in their physical, intellectual, and emotional maturity. At earlier points in time, they will have more undeveloped language, cognitive, and coping skills, and these should become more differentiated and advanced, with time approximating the experience and abilities of adults. For example, the baby in the painting of Sam's community will not verbalize to an examiner that she is wanting for food or attention by the mother, but other objective clues will be required to discern this, such as poor weight gain and growth, apathy to the environment, irritability, low interest in play, inability to be consoled, and failure to demonstrate age appropriate milestones (e.g., reaching for objects in the environment and sitting up alone) (McLean & Price 2011). A health care worker charged with evaluating a child also needs to have an adequate familiarity with normal development in children at different ages, as well as the most commonly encountered mental health problems at these ages.

Reliable sources for comprehension information on child development along the major axes of physical, social-emotional, and cognitive-language development are the Zero to Three Organization (Zero to Three 2014) and the Centers for Disease Control parenting series (CDC 2014a).

Populations with special concerns

Here we will apply the developmental perspective to two young populations encountered all too often on the world stage.

Orphans in institutional care: altered early childhood development

The major developmental tasks of early childhood consist of physically controlling one's body and being mobile, understanding the environment and forming relationships with other people facilitated by the secure attachment to a loving parent, and communicating effectively through language (Ollson 2011; Feigelman 2011c, 2011e, 2011d). These tasks require safety, healthy amounts of stimulation, a predictable routine and environment, and a stable primary caregiver.

The AIDS epidemic in many parts of Africa, Asia, and elsewhere has left behind skyrocketing numbers of orphans (USAID 2014). While family care, foster care, and adoption is encouraged, the high cost of these interventions and at times family level stigma against the children mean that most orphans are still cared for in large institutional centers, raising concerns invoked by the orphanages of prior generations where extreme deprivation and under-stimulation were rampant (Kumar 2012). Social stigma remains a serious problem for these children, who live in shame for the actions of their deceased parents (Deacon & Stephney 2007). The unfortunate mental health outcomes of these circumstances include brain neural circuits negatively affected by chronic stress, attachment problems, and long-term impairments in cognition and language (Pollak et al. 2010).

The child soldier: the hijacking of mid–late childhood and adolescence

Although hardly a new group, child soldiers have been receiving increased attention for the especially challenging social mental health issues they pose. The creation of a child soldier completely undermines and destroys important achievements of middle to late childhood and adolescence. These achievements include sublimation of urges from earlier childhood; empathy and morality; development of confidence and self-esteem; the cultivation of interests; the ability to engage in healthy competition and healthy friendships; sexual maturation and interest in intimate relationships; an evolving relationship with parents that includes a healthy separation and individuation; and the development of higher order cognitive abilities and abstract thinking (Feigelman 2011b; Cromer 2011). Child soldiering distorts and manipulates the adolescent desire to form their own social groups, ruptures a child's relationship with his or her family and natural environment, abruptly puts an end to formal schooling, and encourages aggression (physical, sexual, emotional types) as a way of managing conflict. The 'better' cases are merely threatened and coerced into conscription to serve in domestic and supportive roles, but in worst-case scenarios they are kidnapped and brutalized into participating in armed combat. Child soldiers are often both perpetrators and victim/survivors of the most horrific atrocities against those they love and grew up with, and in some cases do not fully appreciate the gravity of what they have done until much later when it is too late. The traumas to which they are exposed span committing and witnessing murders, rape, torture and physical abuse, losing limbs or sustaining serious physical injuries from detonated mines and weaponry, and needing drug and alcohol abuse as a coping strategy. If they are lucky enough to be released or rescued, they frequently face a grim future, owing to rejection and stigmatization by their families and communities for what they have done (Stevens 2014). The unfortunate psychiatric consequence of these horrific experiences often is a phenomenon known as complex PTSD. This disorder includes problems of alteration between rage and affective emptiness, risky behavior, memory and attention problems, perceiving self as damaged, feeling guilt and shame, possessing an inability to trust, somatization, and loss of faith/hopelessness (Herman, 1992).

A word on epidemiology

As noted in Chapter 1, it is difficult to appreciate the breadth and scope of child mental health disorders on a global scale as comprehensive data is lacking in this regard. Some child epidemiologic data is available for developed countries, but not to the same extent as for adult disorders as described in Chapter 1. In 2005, a 10-year review of prevalence studies for child psychiatric disorders in the US and the UK was published, and the median prevalence estimates of various mental disorders were summarized (Costello et al. 2005). Overall, the median prevalence estimate of functionally impairing child and adolescent psychiatric disorders was 12 percent, with a wide range noted. Among the specific mental disorders, the top four mental disorders in children ages 5–17 included any anxiety disorder, disruptive behavior disorders, major depression, and substance abuse/dependence (Costello et al. 2005). Suicide in younger people also remains a major public health concern: in the US, it is the third leading cause of death in those aged 10–24, and worldwide, among 15–19-year-olds, it is similarly ranked as the leading cause of death (4th for males, 3rd for females) (Wasserman et al. 2005; CDC 2007).

How these estimates correlate to the prevalence of disorders in developing countries and across cultures remains unclear. Nonetheless, if there is any correlation, significant treatment gaps are anticipated, and seriously disabling conditions may be under-recognized and undertreated on the global front.

Evaluation, interventions, and treatment options

Evaluation

Assessment of a child referred for mental health intervention includes inquiry about the nature and duration of the presenting problem, age at first presentation, and associated characteristics of the problem. Next required is a thorough review of prenatal and birth history, especially details about the mother's pregnancy and general state of physical and emotional health, early developmental milestones, temperament (e.g., 'easy or difficult baby'). Next in the history is the family and environmental context of the child's life, family history of mental disorders including substance abuse and suicide. History of trauma is important to inquire about—head injury, abuse (including physical, sexual, emotional types), witnessing or experiencing traumatic events. A history of medical problems, surgeries, and/or injuries is necessary. In addition, the following are important: educational history, problems encountered with learning or academic performance, need for specialized education (if available), individual drug and alcohol history, social history including friendships, interests/hobbies, future goals and wishes, problems with the law/criminal or antisocial behavior (Bostic & King 2007; Gilliam & Mayers 2007).

With regards to identifying specific types of disorders in children, this chapter provides only a brief introduction to working with children and not the detailed approach in diagnosis and assessment that a comprehensive clinical manual would offer. However, a brief review of common childhood mental disorders by age is laid out here for the reader. In the infancy-toddler period, disorders of attachment and development (motor, speech, cognitive delays, intellectual disability, Autism Spectrum Disorders) and failure to thrive are most often encountered (Gilliam & Mayers 2007). In the preschool to young school age years the problems encountered include ADHD (a problem of hyperactivity, impulsiveness, disorganization and/or inattention) and other disruptive behaviors, problems with self-regulation such as prolonged tantrumming and aggression, disorders of speech and language, and anxiety around separation. Disorders of the elementary (primary) school age child will often present as separation issues and somatic expression of anxiety and distress (e.g. stomach aches), and sometimes specific anxieties around animals/objects (specific phobias), ADHD, disruptive behaviors that are evolving into conduct problems (defiance, bullying, aggressive behavior), speech problems, and learning problems. Older school age children may present with anxiety, school avoidance, obsessive compulsive disorder (OCD), bullying, disruptive behaviors and ADHD, conduct problems including truancy and delinquency with aggression, academic problems including learning disorders, and depression (Bostic & King 2007). Adolescents often present with depression that may lead to suicidality, anxiety that may include panic attacks, academic problems, conduct problems as mentioned above for older children, and substance abuse (Bostic & King 2007). Bipolar disorder and schizophrenia may present in adolescence (possible at earlier childhood stages, but rare) (Birmaher et al. 2007; Gogtay & Rapoport 2007). Abuse, trauma, and post-traumatic stress with PTSD unfortunately occur at all stages of childhood, though they are most recognizable in older children and adolescents (Cohen et al. 2010). For a good primer on the 'how-to' aspect of detecting mental health problems in children (as well as adults) we refer you to the book, *Where There is no Psychiatrist: A Mental Health Care Manual* by Vikram Patel (2003).

Interventions and treatment options

Prevention of mental disorders is paramount; helping children avoid circumstances that put them at risk for illness and impairment can mitigate the severity of or possibly eliminate the onset and appearance of future conditions. Community level prevention includes education and awareness about how to maintain child and family health through nutrition/health care/public safety campaigns, reduce stigma around mental health problems and substance abuse, how to foster healthy development, how to recognize impairments in children and adults, how to seek help for mental health issues, reduce/eliminate domestic violence and child abuse. The venues and vehicles for much of the education and awareness efforts towards these public health goals could include local religious and social-cultural institutions. A well-functioning school system with informed teachers and staff also plays an immensely valuable role promoting normal child development and mental health by providing much needed education but also by providing structure, routines, and support from peers and adults (Belfer & Eisenbruch 2007).

Interventions can be applied at one or more of the three levels impacting children—community, family, and individual, and optimally, will include all of them. Psycho-education is an important component of the mental health provider's toolbox (Boettcher & Piacentini 2007). Helping communities, especially teachers and other adults, along with family members and the children themselves understand the mental disorders that afflict children and their families is important in recovery process, and, in the case of episodic and recurrent illnesses such as depression and bipolar disorders, relapse prevention (Birmaher et al. 2007; Birmaher & Brent, 2007).

Parent training is a valuable intervention method in child mental health treatment. The goals of parent training are to support and help parents master basic parenting skills as well as manage more complicated child behavior problems in the home. This can include specialized planning such as using token economy or other behavioral management plans using rewards and consequences for behavioral problems associated with ADHD, disruptive behaviors, and conduct problems. Parent support groups are also valuable in providing peer support for families facing serious mental health challenges with their children.

Schools are an important place for mental health intervention. This includes the need for evaluation and specialized educational programming for children with cognitive delays and problems with academic performance/learning, which when unaddressed, can lead to behavioral problems and distress. Low resource settings will find providing such resource intense education to be a challenge, but problems such as ADHD and disruptive behaviors can at least be addressed via teacher training on behavioral management (Boettcher & Piacentini 2007).

Psychosocial rehabilitation and social skills training are important modalities in pediatric mental health that teach social and communication skills to children that have impairments in these areas (Thienemann 2009). These approaches can be implemented at the level of family and schools. Organized recreation and sports for children such as clubs, youth groups, and sports leagues can play a vital role in psychosocial rehabilitation and social skills training. Finally, play of all kinds—whether in the form of sports, imaginative play with toys, dolls, and other figures—is an essential need for all children. Children use play to amuse themselves, but also, more importantly, to express their inner life in a way that is familiar and safe to them, without the need of advanced language or even cognitive ability and without the direction of adults. Even the most emotionally damaged child has the ability to play, and for children with mental disorders, play can have tremendous therapeutic value. Store bought toys or sports equipment are not even required for children to play—children have the ability, if allowed and encouraged by the adults, to fashion toys out of virtually any material (e.g., corn husks become dolls, cast off wire and trash become pretend vehicles, a fallen melon or a mango become footballs)!

There are a range of psychotherapies available to address childhood disorders. Such therapies are useful in the treatments of depression, anxiety, and traumatic stress, as well as other problems. Individual, family, and group versions of some of these therapies exist. The specific therapies include cognitive-behavioral psychotherapy (CBT), which addresses dysfunctional ways of thinking about one's self and the world and related behaviors; a specialized version of CBT, trauma-focused CBT (TF-CBT), which applies to the treatment of post-traumatic stress using CBT methodology; and interpersonal psychotherapy (IPT), which specifically helps children/adolescents overcome depression by understanding the impact of relationships on how they are feeling (Boettcher & Piacentini 2007; Mufson & Young 2007). Older children and adolescents are best suited to CBT and IPT. Infants and younger children can be therapeutically engaged using psychodynamic play therapy, where toys and imaginative play are used as a means to help master conflicts and anxieties.

There is abundant reason to think these therapies should apply across diverse cultures and communities. But the research to show for it is only emerging: a small randomized control trial (RCT) with 50 boys in the Democratic Republic of Congo found that a culturally modified, group-based TF-CBT intervention was effective in reducing post-traumatic stress and psychosocial distress in former child soldiers and other war-affected boys (McMullen et al. 2013). Another RCT involving 85 former Ugandan child soldiers showed that short-term trauma-focused treatment compared either with an academic catch-up program including supportive counseling or with wait-listing resulted in greater reduction of PTSD symptoms (Ertl et al. 2011).

Medications

Pediatric psychopharmacology is a highly specialized practice, and largely falls beyond the scope of a single chapter on children. The reader may wish to consult further guidelines on practice available through professional resources such as the Practice Parameters issued by the American Academy of Child and Adolescent Psychiatry (AACAP 2014). Nonetheless, there is a need to be mindful in general about the role of medications in the treatment of childhood emotional and behavioral disturbance, as it is somewhat different from that of adults and more complex for several reasons.

Reason 1: because they are such an intimate part of the family and community system, treatment of a child's mental health disorder is highly dependent upon the participation of primary caregivers and other external elements (e.g. teachers and school, extended circle of adult caregivers, siblings and peers, routine and environment) in the child's life. Medication is but one piece in the context of a child's larger treatment efforts. In fact, engagement of these other aspects of a child life along with the use of non-pharmacologic methods at the level of the individual can be so powerful in the child's recovery from distress and disorder, that such efforts alone may reduce or eliminate the need for medications entirely (Boettcher & Piacentini 2007).

Reason 2: the placebo response for some medications and conditions in children is very high compared to the counterpart adult situation (e.g., antidepressants and adolescent depression), supporting the possibility that other factors outside of medication are important in symptom reduction (Cohen et al. 2008).

Reason 3: some psychoactive drugs have robust evidence to support their use in adults but have failed to show the same benefit in children, and in fact can be problematic or hazardous in children. This is the case for benzodiazepines, which are major agents in treatment of adult anxiety but often discouraged for use in children, particularly younger ones who can experience a paradoxical effect on behavior (more excitable instead of less) and in children with respiratory compromise due to risk of respiratory suppression (Connolly et al. 2007).

Reason 4: bias and uncertainty exist on the part of parents around the use of certain medications such as the antidepressants, which have been shown to be associated with increased suicidality in youth during the early weeks of treatment and for which advisories have been made for special monitoring (Bridge et al. 2007). Sadly, since the 'black box' warnings about suicide risk were issued, pediatric prescribing rates in the US have dropped, suicide rates are up, and new risks are posed for the under-treatment of clinical depression in the US community (Lu et al. 2014).

Reason 5: some illnesses are harder to recognize and treat in children compared to adults. An example of such includes the pediatric presentation of psychosis, where a child's language and cognitive development may preclude her from describing delusions or acknowledging hallucinations, but instead, exhibit nonspecific but bizarre, disruptive, and aggressive behavior (McClellan et al. 2013).

Reason 6: less formal approval exists for the use of psychoactive medications in children even in developed countries, and as a result, pharmacotherapy is more challenging in children. The Food and Drug Administration (FDA) in the US, and Medicines and Healthcare products Regulatory Agency (MHRA) in the UK, are charged with providing official approval for medicines in the pediatric population. Unfortunately, far fewer clinical trials and more limited studies in children exist for most psychiatric medications, and less approvals are issued for children overall. As a result, practitioners who are comfortable doing so must often prescribe medications 'off label' (treatment that is probably safe and judicious, but without the formal approval by the regulatory agencies) for a variety of psychiatric conditions in children.

Reason 7: there exists much hesitation around prescribing psychoactive medications to children due to assumptions that harm will be done to the growing brain. This is the case for prenatal exposures to some agents—many antiepileptic medicines can cause neural tube defects (Yerby 2003). However, the example of antidepressants challenges the general belief that children's brains are harmed by medication treatment, as no data supports the notion that antidepressants have a detrimental effect on behavior or neurodevelopment when given to children or adolescents. In fact, emerging evidence supports the argument that treatment of depression during childhood and adolescence restores healthy brain development (Cullen et al. 2009).

The WHO List of Essential Medications (MLEM) as reviewed in Chapters 2 and 5 speaks about the psychoactive medications that should be available to adults in need of pharmacotherapy (WHO 2013). An even more limited list for children under 12 is also available. Just a few comments will be offered on this subject. All classes of agents, whether on the adult or child list, warrant consideration with children as many of the agents have been shown to have therapeutic value with children in research and clinical settings in developed countries (Walkup & the AACAP Work Group on Quality Issues 2009). The atypical antipsychotic medications of risperidone and clozapine are two such examples valued in the treatment of such problems as aggression, treatment refractory psychosis and bipolar disorders (Findling et al. 2011). Another important consideration for children from the list is fluoxetine, as it is the most widely studied agent effective in pediatric depression and the class of medicines (the SSRIs) that are the preferred pharmacologic agent in the treatment of pediatric anxiety (Connolly et al. 2007; Birmaher et al. 2007).

This brings us to a serious omission in the MLEM of stimulant medications, given the 6 percent prevalence of ADHD in the pediatric population (Polanczyk et al. 2007) and evidence that speaks to the use of medication alone or in combination with intensive behavioral treatments as highly effective therapy for ADHD in children (MTA Cooperative Group 1999). The reasons for this continued omission may be related to concerns that stimulant medications are frequently abused, have market value on the street, and, in countries that allow them, require a higher level of regulation unavailable in developing countries (INCSR 2013). It remains hard to reconcile, though that the WHO mhGAP Intervention Guide would give recommendations and detailed instruction on the dosing of methylphenidate for ADHD in children, and yet leave it off its own MLEM (WHO 2010).

Conclusions

Addressing global child mental health requires mindfulness of the child as a part of community, family, and as an individual. It also demands an approach that is developmentally informed according to the stage of the child as well as an appreciation of common problems encountered at different ages. Children in resource poor communities face serious challenges, and complex mental health issues raised by war and rampant disease continue to plague much of the world's children. Research and clinical care for these various mental health problems in children continue to lag behind in the developing world. However, a variety of interventions and treatments are potentially available, provided ways to introduce them into local health care systems can be identified.

It is challenging to conclude such an overflowing chapter with a checklist of recommendations, and so we leave you with this:

✓ In addressing child mental health needs around the globe, remember that children are in all respects not just small adults!

Note

1 While child specialists are often well aware and attuned to the unique developmental status of infants and adolescents, for the purpose of this chapter, the term 'child' and 'children' will be used broadly, keeping with the UN convention, unless stage specific characteristics are being discussed, at which time the terms 'infant,' 'baby,' 'adolescent,' or 'teenager' will be used.

References

AACAP 2014, *Practice Parameters*. Available: www.aacap.org/AACAP/Resources_for_Primary_Care/Practice_Parameters_and_Resource_Centers/Practice_Parameters1.aspx (accessed September 28, 2014).

Albee, G.W. 1986, 'Toward a just society. Lessons on the primary prevention of psychopathology,' *American Psychologist*, vol. 41, no. 8, pp. 891–898.

American Psychiatric Association 2013, *Diagnostic and Statistical Manual of Mental Disorders, Fifth Edition (DSM 5)*, American Psychiatric Association, Washington, D.C.

Aristophanes 423BC, 'Children should be seen and not heard,' *The Clouds*, I. 963, in B. Stevenson 1949, *B. Stevenson's Book of Proverbs, Maxims and Familiar Phrases*, Routledge and Kegan Paul Ltd, London.

Belfer, M. & Eisenbruch, M. 2007, 'International child and adolescent mental health,' in A. Martin & F.R. Volkmar (eds.), *Lewis's Child and Adolescent Psychiatry: A Comprehensive Textbook*, 4th Edition, Lippincott Williams & Wilkins, Philadelphia, Chapter 1.8.

Betancourt, T.S. 2010, 'Past horrors, present struggles: the role of stigma in the association between war experiences and psychosocial adjustment among former child soldiers in Sierra Leone,' *Social Science & Medicine*, vol. 7, no. 1, pp. 17–26.

Birmaher, B. & Brent, D. (AACAP Work Group on Quality Issues) 2007, 'Practice parameter for the assessment and treatment of children and adolescents with depressive disorders,' *Journal of the American Academy of Child and Adolescent Psychiatry*, vol. 46, no. 11, pp. 1503–1526.

Birmaher, B., Axelson, D., & Pavuluri, M. 2007, 'Bipolar disorder,' in A. Martin & F.R. Volkmar (eds.), *Lewis's Child and Adolescent Psychiatry: A Comprehensive Textbook*, 4th Edition, Lippincott Williams & Wilkins, Philadelphia, Chapter 5.4.2.

Boettcher, M.A. & Piacentini, J. 2007, 'Cognitive and behavioral therapies,' in A. Martin & F.R. Volkmar (eds.), *Lewis's Child and Adolescent Psychiatry: A Comprehensive Textbook*, 4th Edition, Lippincott Williams & Wilkins, Philadelphia, Chapter 6.2.2.

Bostic, J.Q. & King, R.A. 2007. 'Clinical assessment of children and adolescents: content and structure,' in A. Martin & F.R. Volkmar (eds.), *Lewis's Child and Adolescent Psychiatry: A Comprehensive Textbook*, 4th Edition, Lippincott Williams & Wilkins, Philadelphia, Chapter 4.2.2.

Bowlby, J. 1980, *Attachment and Loss: Volume III: Loss, Sadness, and Depression*, The Hogarth Press and the Institute for Psychoanalysis, London, The International Psychoanalytic Library, vol. 109, pp. 1–462.

Bridge, J.A., Iyengar, S., Salary, C.B., Barbe, R.P., Birmaher, B., Pincus, H.A., Ren, L., & Brent, D.A. 2007, 'Clinical response and risk for reported suicidal ideation and suicide attempts in pediatric antidepressant treatment: a meta-analysis of randomized controlled trials,' *Journal of the American Medical Association*, vol. 297, pp. 1683–1696.

CDC 2014a, *Development and Positive Parenting Series*. Available: www.cdc.gov/ncbddd/childdevelopment/positiveparenting/ (accessed September 29, 2014).

CDC 2014b, *Fact Sheet on the Impact of Malaria*. Available: www.cdc.gov/malaria/malaria_worldwide/impact.html (accessed September 28, 2014).

Centers for Disease Control and Prevention 2007, 'Suicide trends among youths and young adults aged 10–24 years—United States, 1990–2004,' *MMWR Morbidity and Mortality Weekly Report*, vol. 56, no. 35, pp. 905–908.

Cohen, D., Deniau, E., Maturana, A., Tanguy, M.L., Bodeau, N., Labelle, R., Breton, J.J., & Guile, J.M. 2008, 'Are child and adolescent responses to placebo higher in major depression than in anxiety disorders? A systematic review of placebo-controlled trials,' *PLoS One*, vol. 3, no. 7, p. e2632, doi:10.1371/journal.pone.0002632.

Cohen, J.A. and AACAP the Work Group on Quality Issues, 2010. 'Practice parameter for the assessment and treatment of children and adolescents with post traumatic stress disorder,' *Journal of the American Academy of Child & Adolescent Psychiatry*, vol. 37, no. 10, Suppl. pp. 4S–26S.

Collins, P.Y., Patel, V., Joestl, S.S., March, D., Insel, T.R., Daar, A.S., Scientific Advisory Board and the Executive Committee of the Grand Challenges on Global Mental Health et al. 2011, 'Grand challenges in global mental health,' *Nature*, vol. 475, no. 7354, pp. 27–30.

Connolly, S.D., Bernstein G.A., & Work Group on Quality Issues 2007, 'Practice parameter for the assessment and treatment of children and adolescents with anxiety disorders,' *Journal of the American Academy of Child and Adolescent Psychiatry*, vol. 46, no. 2, pp. 267–283.

Costello, E., Egger, H., & Angold, A. 2005, '10-year research update review: the epidemiology of child and adolescent psychiatric disorders: I. Methods and public health burden,' *Journal of the American Academy Child and Adolescent Psychiatry*, vol. 44, no. 10, pp. 972–986.

Cromer, B. 2011, 'Adolescent physical and social development,' in R.G. Kliegman, B.F. Stanton, J.W. St. Geme III, N.F. Schor, & R.E. Behrman (eds.), *Nelson Textbook of Pediatrics*, 19th Edition, Elsevier Saunders Inc., Philadelphia, pp. 649–659.e1.

Cullen, K., Klimes-Dougan, B., & Kumra, S. 2009, 'Pediatric depression: issues and treatment recommendations,' *Minnesota Medicine*, vol. 92, no. 3, pp. 45–48.

Deacon, H. & Stephney, I. 2007, *HIV/AIDS, Stigma and Children: A Literature Review*, Human Sciences Research Council, HSRC Press, South Africa, pp. 1–81. Available: www.unaids.org.cn/pics/20120821112026.pdf (accessed October 26, 2014).

Emerson, E. & Einfeld, S. 2010, 'Emotional and behavioural difficulties in young children with and without developmental delay: a bi-national perspective,' *Journal of Child Psychology and Psychiatry*, vol. 51, no. 5, pp. 583–593.

Ertl, V., Pfeiffer, A., Schauer, E., Elbert, T., & Neuner, F. 2011, 'Community-implemented trauma therapy for former child soldiers in Northern Uganda: a randomized controlled trial,' *Journal of the American Medical Association*, vol. 306, no. 5, pp. 503–512.

Esposito, G., Venuti, P., & Bornstein, M.H. 2011, 'Assessment of distress in young children: a comparison of autistic disorder, developmental delay, and typical development,' *Research in Autism Spectrum Disorders*, vol. 5, no. 4, pp. 1510–1516.

Fazel, M. & Stein, A. 2002, 'The mental health of refugee children,' *Archives of Diseases in Children*, vol. 87, pp. 366–370.

Feigelman, S. 2011a, 'Assessment of fetal growth and development,' in R.G. Kliegman, B.F. Stanton, J.W. St. Geme III, N.F. Schor, & R.E. Behrman (eds.), *Nelson Textbook of Pediatrics*, 19th Edition, Elsevier Saunders Inc., Philadelphia, p. 26.e9.

Feigelman, S. 2011b, 'Middle childhood,' in R.G. Kliegman, B.F. Stanton, J.W. St. Geme III, N.F. Schor, & R.E. Behrman (eds.), *Nelson Textbook of Pediatrics*, 19th Edition, Elsevier Saunders Inc., Philadelphia, pp. 36–39.e1.

Feigelman, S. 2011c, 'The first year,' in R.G. Kliegman, B.F. Stanton, J.W. St. Geme III, N.F. Schor, & R.E. Behrman (eds.), *Nelson Textbook of Pediatrics*, 19th Edition, Elsevier Saunders Inc., Philadelphia, pp. 26–31.e1.

Feigelman, S. 2011d, 'The preschool years,' in R.G. Kliegman, B.F. Stanton, J.W. St. Geme III, N.F. Schor, & R.E. Behrman (eds.), *Nelson Textbook of Pediatrics*, 19th Edition, Elsevier Saunders Inc., Philadelphia, pp. 33–36.e1.

Feigelman, S. 2011e, 'The second year,' in R.G. Kliegman, B.F. Stanton, J.W. St. Geme III, N.F. Schor, & R.E. Behrman (eds.), *Nelson Textbook of Pediatrics*, 19th Edition, Elsevier Saunders Inc., Philadelphia, pp. 31–33.e1.

Findling, R.F., Drury, S.S., Jensen, P.S., Rapoport, J.L., and the AACAP Committee on Quality Issues. 2011, *Practice Parameter for the Use of Atypical Antipsychotic Medications in Children and Adolescents*. Available: www.aacap.org/App_Themes/AACAP/docs/practice_parameters/Atypical_Antipsychotic_Medications_Web.pdf (accessed October 27, 2014), pp. 1–27.

Gilliam, W.S. & Mayes, L.C. 2007, 'Clinical assessment of infants and toddlers,' in A. Martin & F.R. Volkmar (eds.), *Lewis's Child and Adolescent Psychiatry: A Comprehensive Textbook*, 4th Edition, Lippincott Williams & Wilkins, Philadelphia, Chapter 4.2.1.

Gogtay, N. & Rapoport, J. 2007, 'Childhood onset schizophrenia and other early-onset psychotic disorders,' in A. Martin & F.R. Volkmar (eds.), *Lewis's Child and*

Adolescent Psychiatry: A Comprehensive Textbook, 4th Edition, Lippincott Williams & Wilkins, Philadelphia, Chapter 5.3

Herman, J. L. 1992, 'Complex PTSD: a syndrome in survivors of prolonged and repeated trauma,' *Journal of Traumatic Stress*, vol. 5, pp. 377–391.

INSCR 2013, *International Narcotics Control Strategy Report*. Available: www.state.gov/j/inl/rls/nrcrpt/2013/index.htm (accessed October 27, 2014).

Kellmer Pringle, M.L. & Bossio, V. 1960, 'Early, prolonged separation and emotional maladjustment,' *Child Psychology And Psychiatry*, vol. 1, no. 1, pp. 37–48.

Kihara, M., Carter, J.A., & Newton, C.R.J.C. 2006, 'The effect of *Plasmodium falciparum* on cognition: a systematic review,' *Tropical Medicine & International Health*, vol. 11, no. 4, pp. 386–397.

Kumar, A. 2012, 'AIDS orphans and vulnerable children in India: problems, prospects, and concerns,' *Social Work in Public Health*, vol. 27, no. 3, pp. 205–212.

Laor, N. & Wolmer, L. 2007, 'Children exposed to disaster: the role of the mental health professional,' in A. Martin & F.R. Volkmar (eds.), *Lewis's Child and Adolescent Psychiatry: A Comprehensive Textbook*, 4th Edition, Lippincott Williams & Wilkins, Philadelphia, Chapter 5.15.5.

Lu, C.Y., Zhang, F., Lakoma, M.D., Madden, J.M., Rusinak, D., Penfold, R.B., et al. 2014, 'Changes in antidepressant use by young people and suicidal behavior after FDA warnings and media coverage: quasi-experimental study,' *British Medical Journal*, vol. 348, p. 3596.

Masten, A.S., Best, K.M., & Garmezy, N. 1990, 'Resilience and development: contributions from the study of children who overcome adversity,' *Development and Psychopathology*, vol. 2, pp. 425–444.

McClellan, J., Stock, S., & American Academy of Child and Adolescent Psychiatry (AACAP) Committee on Quality Issues (CQI) 2013, 'Practice parameter for the assessment and treatment of children and adolescents with schizophrenia,' *Journal of the American Academy of Child and Adolescent Psychiatry*, vol. 52, no. 9, pp. 976–990.

McLean, H.S. & Price, D.T. 2011, 'Failure to thrive,' in R.G. Kliegman, B.F. Stanton, J.W. St. Geme III, N.F. Schor, & R.E. Behrman (eds.), *Nelson Textbook of Pediatrics*, 19th Edition, Elsevier Saunders Inc., Philadelphia, pp. 147–149.

McMullen, J., O'Callaghan, P., Shannon, C., Black, A., & Eakin, J. 2013, 'Group trauma-focused cognitive-behavioural therapy with former child soldiers and other war-affected boys in the DRCongo: a randomised controlled trial,' *Journal of Child Psychology and Psychiatry*, vol. 54, no. 11, pp. 1231–1241.

Minshew, N.J. & Payton, J.B. 1988, 'New perspectives in autism. Part 2: the differential diagnosis and neurobiology of autism,' *Current Problems in Pediatrics*, vol. 18, no. 11, pp. 618–694.

Morris, J., Belfer, M., Daniels, A., Flisher, A., Ville, L., Lora, A. & Saxena, S. 2011, 'Treated prevalence of and mental health services received by children and adolescents in 42 low-and-middle-income countries,' *Journal of Child Psychology and Psychiatry, and Allied Disciplines*, vol. 52, no. 12, pp. 1239–1246.

Morrow, V. 2004, 'Children's social capital: Implications for health and well-being,' *Health Education*, vol. 104, no. 4, pp. 211–225.

MTA Cooperative Group 1999, 'A 14-month randomized clinical trial of treatment strategies for attention-deficit/hyperactivity disorder (ADHD),' *Archives of General Psychiatry*, vol. 56, pp. 1073–1086.

Mufson, L. & Young, J.F. 2007, 'Interpersonal psychotherapy,' in A. Martin & F.R. Volkmar (eds.), *Lewis's Child and Adolescent Psychiatry: A Comprehensive Textbook*, 4th Edition, Lippincott Williams & Wilkins, Philadelphia, Chapter 6.2.3.

Olsson. J. 2011, 'The newborn,' in R.G. Kliegman, B.F. Stanton, J.W. St. Geme III, N.F. Schor, & R.E. Behrman (eds.), *Nelson Textbook of Pediatrics*, 19th Edition, Elsevier Saunders Inc., Philadelphia, pp. 26–26.e12.

Patel, V. 2003, *Where There Is No Psychiatrist. A Mental Health Care Manual*, Chapter 8: Problems in childhood and adolescence, The Royal College of Psychiatrists, London, pp. 155–187.

Patel, V. & Kleinman, A. 2003, 'Poverty and common mental disorders in developing countries,' *Bulletin of the World Health Organization*, vol. 81, no. 8, p. 611.

Pharoah, P.O. & Connolly, K.J. 1995, 'Iodine and brain development,' *Developmental Medicine & Child Neurology*, vol. 37, no. 8, pp. 744–748.

Polanczyk, G., de Lima, M., Horta, B., Biederman, J., & Rohde, L. 2007, 'The worldwide prevalence of ADHD: a systemic review and metaregression analysis,' *American Journal of Psychiatry*, vol. 164, no. 6, pp. 942–948.

Pollak, S.D., Nelson, C.A., Schlaak, M.F., Roeber, B.J., Wewerka, S.S., Wiik, K.L., et al. 2010, 'Neurodevelopmental effects of early deprivation in postinstitutionalized children,' *Child Development*, vol. 81, no. 1, pp. 224–236.

Prado, E.L. & Dewey, K.G. 2014, 'Nutrition and brain development in early life,' *Nutrition Reviews*, vol. 72, no. 4, pp. 267–284.

Prince, M., Patel, V., Saxena, S., Maj, M., Maselko, J., Phillips, M.R., & Rahman, A. 2007, 'No health without mental health,' *The Lancet*, vol. 370, no. 9590, pp. 859–877.

Prober, C.G. & Dyner, L.L. 2011, 'Central nervous system infections,' in R.G. Kliegman, B.F. Stanton, J.W. St. Geme III, N.F. Schor, & R.E. Behrman (eds.), *Nelson Textbook of Pediatrics*, 19th Edition, Elsevier Saunders Inc., Philadelphia, p. 2095.

Putnam, R., Light, I., Briggs, X.d.S., Rohe, W.M., Vidal, A.C., Hutchinson, J., et al. 2004, 'Using social capital to help integrate planning theory, research and practice: preface,' *Journal of the American Planning Association*, vol. 70, no. 2, pp. 142–192.

Saunders, B.E. & Adams, Z.W. 2014, 'Epidemiology of traumatic experiences in childhood,' in S.J. Cozza, J.A. Cohen, & J.G. Dougherty (eds.), *Child and Adolescent Psychiatric Clinics of North America*, vol. 23, no. 2, pp. 167–184.

Shapiro, B.K. & Batshaw, M.L. 2011, 'Intellectual disability,' in R.G. Kliegman, B.F. Stanton, J.W. St. Geme III, N.F. Schor, & R.E. Behrman (eds.), *Nelson Textbook of Pediatrics*, 19th Edition, Elsevier Saunders Inc., Philadelphia, p. 123.

Stevens A.J. 2014, 'The invisible soldiers: understanding how the life experiences of girl child soldiers impacts upon their health and rehabilitation needs,' *Archives of Disease in Children*, vol. 99, no. 5, pp. 458–462.

Stoddard, Jr., F.J. 2014, 'Outcomes of traumatic exposure,' in S.J. Cozza, J.A. Cohen, & J.G. Dougherty (eds.), *Child and Adolescent Psychiatric Clinics of North America*, vol. 23, no. 2, pp. 243–256.

Sullivan, P.M. & Knutson, J.F. 2000, 'Maltreatment and disabilities: a population-based epidemiological study,' *Child Abuse & Neglect*, vol. 24, no. 10, pp. 1257–1273.

Thienemann, M.L. 2009, 'Group psychotherapy,' in B.J. Sadock, V.A. Sadock, & P. Ruiz (eds.), *Kaplan & Sadock's Comprehensive Textbook of Psychiatry*, 9th Edition, Lippincott Williams & Wilkins, Philadelphia, Chapter 51.4.

UNICEF 2014, *Article 1, Convention of the Rights of the Child*. Available: www.ohchr.org/EN/ProfessionalInterest/Pages/CRC.aspx (accessed September 28, 2014).

USAID 2014, *Orphans and Vulnerable Children Affected by HIV*. Available: www.usaid.gov/what-we-do/global-health/hiv-and-aids/technical-areas/orphans-and-vulnerable-children-affected-hiv (accessed October 26, 2014).

Wachs, T.D., Georgieff, M., Cusick, S., & McEwen, B.S. 2014, 'Issues in the timing of integrated early interventions: contributions from nutrition, neuroscience, and psychological research,' *Annals of the New York Academy of Sciences*, vol. 1308, no. 1, pp. 89–106.

Walker, S.P., Wachs, T.D., Gardner, J.M., Lozoff, B., Wasserman, G.A., Pollitt, E., Carter, J.A., & International Child Development Steering Group 2007, 'Child development: risk factors for adverse outcomes in developing countries,' *The Lancet*, vol. 369, no. 9556, pp. 145–157.

Walkup, J. & the AACAP Work Group on Quality Issues 2009, 'Practice parameter on the use of psychotropic medication in children and adolescents,' *Journal of the American Academy of Child and Adolescent Psychiatry*, vol. 48, no. 9, pp. 961–973.

Wasserman, D., Cheng, Q., & Jiang, G.X. 2005, 'Global suicide rates among young people aged 15–19,' *World Psychiatry*, vol. 4, no. 2, pp. 114–120.

WHO 2010, *2010 mhGAP Intervention Guide*. Available: www.who.int/mental_health/publications/mhGAP_intervention_guide/en/ (accessed September 29, 2014).

WHO 2013, *Essential Medicines 2013*. Available: www.who.int/medicines/services/essmedicines_def/en/ (accessed September 27, 2014).

Yerby, M.S. 2003, 'Clinical care of pregnant women with epilepsy: neural tube defects and folic acid supplementation,' *Epilepsia*, vol. 44, suppl. 3, pp. 33–40.

Zero To Three 2014, National Center for Infants, Toddlers and Families age based handouts for parents. Available: www.zerotothree.org/about-us/areas-of-expertise/free-parent-brochures-and-guides/age-based-handouts.html (accessed September 29, 2014).

Chapter 9

Disasters

Look closely and notice the water line that stretches across the facade of the buildings in the photo. This is a residue of the typhoon that struck the country nearly eight months ago. Before that, the five-year civil war took thousands of lives and displaced even more people. Everyone was affected in some way. It was a war notorious worldwide for the conscription of child soldiers and the inscrutability of its rationale.

Maybe it was the senselessness of it all that permitted the typhoon to effectively wash it away. When it struck, the war had long since become a daily routine, mundane and habitual. The agrarian economy had even re-oriented itself around it, with farmers becoming mercenary soldiers and farms battlegrounds.

The typhoon lashed the country with a powerful jolt that caught people off guard. Mass death at the hands of the gods was too much to bear, and many took it as punishment for the war. A national day of prayer was declared. People flocked to temples and never returned to the battlefield.

With the peace and worldwide media coverage of bodies floating in the streets of the capital, humanitarian aid poured in anew, along with a smattering of global mental health professionals. Like the waterline, infrastructure damage endures to this day. Damage to bridges and roadways has transformed what would have been a three-hour drive for Sam to see his wife and kids to the present day 10-hour journey. No one expects this to be corrected in the near future and possibly even in their lifetimes.

Whether manmade or natural, disasters change the landscape. In the immediate aftermath of disaster, saving lives is the priority. Over the long term, the focus drifts towards restoration of the living environment and rebuilding of infrastructure. Mental health issues stretch out across this timeline from just beyond the time of impact indefinitely into the future. It has in fact been estimated that infrastructure recovery takes 10 times as long as the immediate response efforts and that the timeframe for psychological recovery is incalculably longer (Chandra & Acosta 2010). We will here talk about the mental health dimensions of disasters from both the short and long term perspective and talk about the global mental health professional as a 'disaster mental health professional.'

Reactions to disaster

In the immediate aftermath of a disaster, as with trauma in general, survivors' responses are varied. Many people experience a range of emotions and thoughts as well as potentially dysfunctional behavioral change. Emotionally it can be a 'rollercoaster' of sadness, grief, despair, and fear as well as elation and inspiration. Thoughts can range as far as questioning how to go on in life without loved ones, reflecting powerful existential questions that fortunately rarely cross into suicidality. Concerning behaviors include sleep disturbance and turning to alcohol or drugs to cope (Katz 2011c).

Particularly in non-Western settings like that depicted in this book, a fourth type of reaction should be considered, namely physical complaints whose quality or other features are not consistent with a medical explanation. Unexplained medical symptoms and non-specific symptoms such as headache or dyspepsia are often the way many people and many cultures experience their distress (Van Moffaert 1998; Escobar et al. 1992). It might be said that Westerners tend towards psychologizing whereas non-Westerners tend towards somaticizing. Global mental health professionals are advised not to take psychologizing as the standard to be aspired to.

Overall, many of the acute reactions to disaster are normal and even adaptive. For example, in the uncertain immediate aftermath, not sleeping as much as usual may permit the level of vigilance demanded to monitor the situation. Reactions become symptoms of clinical concern when they are too disruptive, too distressing, too dangerous, or too long lasting, leaving room for much clinical judgment regarding what is pathological. An oft-cited way of looking at it is that most people's reactions to a disaster are 'normal reactions to an abnormal event.' Disasters are not clinical settings and therefore when working in the field in response to a disaster, the presumption tends to be for mental health and normality until proven otherwise. This is especially important in the face of criticisms, sometimes justified and sometimes strident, that mental health professionals' involvement with recent disaster survivors will pathologize their normal responses (Summerfield 2006).

One approach might then be to avoid designating acute traumatic reactions as either symptoms or disorders but rather to borrow from military experience and call them 'stress injuries' and then differentiating these based on the causative agent— trauma, grief, and fatigue (Figley & Nash 2007). However, as this is not standard diagnostic approach, we recommend it as a framework with which global mental health professionals can think about the matter and not as a diagnostic system.

There are well-established risk factors for gauging what immediate reactions are likely to evolve into clinical conditions such as the two most common long-term consequences of disaster, Major Depression and Post-Traumatic Stress Disorder (PTSD). These include the following (Katz 2011a):

- Prior exposure to trauma such as disaster
- Prior psychiatric history
- Problems of living prior to the disaster/low socioeconomic status
- Lack of perceived or actual social supports after the event
- Presence of 'secondary stressors'
- Female
- Middle age
- Ethnic minority.

As an example, when refugees living in a tent city in Turkey after fleeing the ongoing civil war in Syria were recently evaluated by a psychiatrist, PTSD was found in a very high one-third of the sample and was most prevalent among women refugees or those who had a personal or family psychiatric history or who experienced two or more traumas (Alpak et al. 2014).

Post-traumatic risk factors are worth thinking about in the context of Sam and his countrymen. Besides what he witnessed and experienced at the time of the typhoon, Sam just endured the prior trauma of five years of civil war; is living in poverty; lacks social support in the form of a nuclear family; and has the added financial stress of a struggling farming business due to the effects of both flooding and civil war. This constellation of traumatogenic problems is not unrealistic and very common in too many places around the world.

On other hand, there is increasing appreciation for the resiliency that many people demonstrate in the face of trauma. A host of resiliency factors are thought to help insulate people from the traumatic effects of disaster and may even contribute to so-called 'post-traumatic growth.' Here is a comprehensive list (Southwick & Charney 2012):

- Realistic optimism
- Facing fear
- Moral compass
- Religion and spirituality
- Social support
- Resilient role models
- Physical fitness
- Brain fitness
- Cognitive and emotional flexibility
- Meaning and purpose.

Many of these factors are modifiable and can be influenced or nurtured (i.e., cognitive flexibility) by the global mental health professional as well as many other sources. In many countries, religion plays an especially important role in both daily life and times of disaster. We have been struck by how often we have heard people come to terms with catastrophe by explaining it away as 'god's will.' Think also about Sam's stopping in at the faith healer/minister—irrespective of the details of or the scientific evidence for the healer's techniques, the healer at least provides social support and fosters spirituality all at once.

Acute interventions

In a newspaper editorial following the 2004 South Asian tsunami entitled *Bread and Shelters, Yes. Psychiatrists, No*, the writer casts the arrival of mental health professionals into post-tsunami Sri Lanka as well intentioned but misguided (Satel 2005). Her basic point was that what Sri Lankans needed far more than specialized psychiatric services were essentials such as food, shelter, and jobs. In fact, her position runs the risk of creating a paper tiger of 'either/or' choices when in fact concrete needs and disaster psychiatry (and global psychiatry in general—see Chapter 7) are not mutually exclusive and can and should overlap. A psychiatrist who does not appreciate that people need bread and shelter before all else has no more of a place

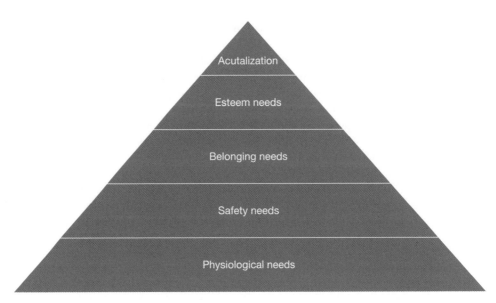

Figure 9.1 Maslow's hierarchy of human needs

on New York's wealthy Park Avenue than in the tsunami zone of South Asia. Even more so in times of disaster than otherwise, there must be a prioritization of people's fundamental human needs. This is best embodied in Maslow's classic hierarchy of human needs, which reminds us that safety and physiological needs come before all else (Maslow 1943) (Figure 9.1).

Once the global mental health practitioner has assured that such needs have been addressed sufficiently, whether through their own efforts or those of others, it is possible to move unto the higher order needs that are typically more associated with the purview of mental health professionals—belonging, esteem, and actualization. Of course, if in the usual states of affairs in countries like Sam's there is shortage of human and non-human mental health resources (see Chapters 2 and 3), this is sure to be exacerbated right after a disaster. On the other hand, the eventual influx of foreign aid can at least reverse shortages of psychiatric supplies if not temporarily enhance pre-event levels. However, the likelihood of aid agencies incorporating mental health into their response will be very low unless global mental health professionals (as well as mental health professional associations) advocate for this, ideally in advance of crises (see Chapter 4 for a further discussion of advocacy and activism).

Further, the scant evidence base to inform mental health interventions with recently traumatized individuals makes helping disaster survivors a challenge in any setting irrespective of its income level (Katz 2011b). Fortunately, there is at least an evidence informed framework for intervening with recent survivors known as psychological first aid or PFA (Kantor & Beckert 2011). Importantly for already low resource settings, PFA can be practiced by non-mental health professionals, and even in many cases non-health professionals, given that it also relies on many factors that are intuitive, cost-effective, and non-technical.

The major Maslow-like tenets of PFA are as follows (Brymer et al. 2006):

- Contact and engage survivors.
- Ensure safety and comfort.
- Stabilize those in most distress.
- Identify current needs and concerns.
- Assist with practical needs.
- Connect with social supports.
- Provide psychoeducation on coping after trauma.
- Orient and connect to available services.

PFA establishes a broad framework in which simple human connection and engagement, practical assistance, education, linkage with family and friends, and referral to relief agencies have a place in the toolkit of the disaster mental health responder. This framework is also flexible enough to permit judicious use of explicitly psychiatric interventions such as acute psychotropic use and psychotherapy. An example of the former would be short term prescription of a medicine such as diazepam that is likely available in most any setting to someone in acute distress. Common sense and experience both suggest that PFA can be applied cross-culturally (Brymer et al. 2006). For example, we are aware of its extensive use in Japan after the earthquake/tsunami/radiation disaster of March 2011.

Finally, there is a child/adolescent version of PFA (Schreiber & Gurwich 2006). It rests on the three essential principles of 'listen, protect, and connect' as a guide for parents and other child caretakers, as follows:

1 *Listen* and pay attention to what children say and how they act.
2 *Protect* children by way of sharing information about the disaster and about the measures being taken to keep them safe.
3 *Connect* children with family, friends, schoolmates, teachers, and others as soon as is feasible.

Long term interventions

Mental health care generally consists of long term efforts, and disaster mental health care is much the same. Although most people will typically see their acute symptoms (or 'stress injuries') resolve with time and with little or no professional assistance, some people who meet even part of the risk profile described earlier will go on to have long term mental health problems. Disaster mental health professionals can be helpful in the acute aftermath but also can play a role in the long term when the world's attention fades (Katz 2013).

Involvement in the long term affords the chance and privilege to help a community get back to a 'new normal.' It is also may permit re-building of a more vibrant mental health system than was there before the event due to the influx of funding and the political will generated by disasters. Disaster mental health professionals should avoid being 'disaster tourists' who rush in amid media attention never to be seen again—disaster mental health tourists not only benefit themselves more than the community of concern but also risk damaging the already tenuous reputation of their field of mental health.

Clinical guidance

We suggest 'The Three W's' as a clinical framework for assessing and addressing post-disaster mental health needs (Disaster Psychiatry Outreach 2004). The three W's are: *what* is known about the event; *who* is the person being evaluated; and *when* in the aftermath of the disaster are they being evaluated?

What is known about the event, including its scope, impact, and public health implications?

a   Impact of disaster—injured, dead, exposed, displaced, unemployed
b   Information about the affected community's *pre-event* public health/mental health, social, political, and economic functioning.
c   Unique psychological themes for the type of event, e.g. earthquakes, aviation disasters, terrorist events.

Who is the person under consideration, including their personal, social, and psychological history as well as their connection to the disaster?

a   Demographics—age, gender, marital status, employment, living situation
b   Psychological responses
c   Exposure
d   Role in the 'disaster community' that rises up around an event
e   Presence of other risk factors for psychological problems
f   Resources (e.g., family, friends, relatives)
g   Culture

When in the time course of the event are they being seen?

a   Impact (minutes to hours to days)—application of PFA by provision of basic empathy, support, orientation, accurate information, structure and direction to the experience.
b   Acute phase (days to weeks)—evaluating for biopsychosocial needs, distress responses, behavioral changes, risk factors, personal meaning, and resiliency.
c   Post-acute phase (weeks to months to years)—evaluating for psychiatric illness as well as biopsychosocial needs, risk factors, personal meaning, and resiliency.

Application of these three questions will help to create a three-dimensional view of the survivor and their community. They will also orient the disaster mental health practitioner to the timeframe and the psychological consequences appropriate for consideration.

Conclusions

Many mental health professionals feel the pull of global work in particular during times of disaster. If you decide to work in a disaster and have not done so before, please keep things in perspective. Disaster stricken communities around the world had a pre-event identity and needs and will again return to a normal footing when the huge unmet mental health needs of normal life that we discussed in Chapter 1 will still abound. In fact, among the survivors most at risk for long term mental health problems are those very ones who had pre-disaster mental health problems. There is therefore an argument to be made that participating in global mental health work in disaster-free times and thereby making a country or community or people mentally healthy better positions them to thrive in daily life and in the rare event of a disaster (Katz 2011b).

Here we leave you with some final considerations about your work as a disaster mental health professional:

✓ Remember that in the acute aftermath of a disaster, you should consider yourself a humanitarian first, a doctor or health/public health professional second, and a global mental health professional third. If you do not think you can abide by this hierarchy, you should re-consider going.

✓ If you function as a mental health clinician in the immediate wake of a disaster, think symptoms or even 'stress injuries' and not disorders. Beware pathologizing, as disorders usually come later.

✓ But, do not just think symptoms or stress injuries, as people have much on their minds. Think psychology. For example, instead of just inquiring about someone's sleep, ask also about what is on their mind when they lay awake at night.

✓ In the spirit of mental health in general, Psychological First Aid, and common humanity, listen to the people you are helping. Many cultures do not endorse 'opening up' the way much of the developed world does, but we find that people inevitably open up in healthy ways when given private space and a kind ear.

✓ If you cannot remember the principles of PFA or even want to enrich them, remember these five overarching principles (Duckers 2013):

  ✓ Promote a sense of safety.
  ✓ Promote calming.
  ✓ Promote sense of self and collective efficacy.
  ✓ Promote connectedness.
  ✓ Promote hope.

✓ Finally, consider disasters opportunities to make things better than they were before, as the pre-disaster story of many localities is often a sad one. In fact, it is the most vulnerable communities which suffer the most from disasters. Post-disaster periods are highly dynamic times well suited to advocacy and activism by interested global mental health professionals.

References

Alpak, G., Unal, A., Bulbul, F., Salgatici, E., Bez, Y., Altindag, A., et al. 2014. 'Post-traumatic stress disorder among Syrian refugees in Turkey: a cross-sectional study,' *International Journal of Psychiatry in Clinical Practice*, doi: 10.3109/136511501.2014.961930.

Brymer, M., Jacobs, A., Layne, C., Pynoos, R., Ruzek, J., Steinberg, A., et al. 2006, *Psychological First Aid: Field Operations Guide, 2nd Edition*. Available: www.ptsd.va.gov/professional/materials/manuals/psych-first-aid.asp (accessed January 23, 2014).

Chandra, A. & Acosta, J.D. 2010, 'Disaster recovery also involves human recovery,' *JAMA: The Journal of the American Medical Association*, vol. 304, no. 14, pp. 1608–1609.

Disaster Psychiatry Outreach 2004, *Mental Health Consequences of Bioterrorism: A Disaster Preparedness Course for Hospital Emergency Department Staff*. Training Course edn, Health Resources and Services Administration (Grant Number U3RMC01549-01).

Duckers, M.L. 2013, 'Five essential principles of post-disaster psychosocial care: looking back and forward with Stevan Hobfoll,' *European Journal of Psychotraumatology*, vol. 4, pp. 10.3402/ejpt.v4i0.21914.

Escobar, J.I., Canino, G., Rubio-Stipec, M., & Bravo, M. 1992, 'Somatic symptoms after a natural disaster: a prospective study,' *American Journal of Psychiatry*, vol. 149, pp. 965–967.

Figley, C.R. & Nash, W.P. 2007, *Combat Stress Injury*, Brunner-Routledge, New York.

Kantor, E. & Beckert, D. 2011, 'Psychological first aid' in F. Stoddard, A. Pandya, & C. Katz (eds.), *Disaster Psychiatry: Readiness, Evaluation, and Treatment*, American Psychiatric Press, Inc., Washington, D.C., pp. 203–212.

Katz, C. 2011a, 'Psychiatric evaluation' in F. Stoddard, A. Pandya, & C.L. Katz (eds.), *Clinical Manual of Disaster Psychiatry*, American Psychiatric Press, Arlington, VA, pp. 71–88.

Katz, C.L. 2011b, 'Disaster psychiatry: good intentions seeking science and sustainability,' *Adolescent Psychiatry*, vol. 1, no. 3, pp. 187–196.

Katz, C.L. 2011c, 'Psychiatric evaluation' in F. Stoddard, A. Pandya, & C. Katz (eds.), *Disaster Psychiatry: Readiness, Evaluation, and Treatment*, American Psychiatric Press, Inc., Washington, D.C., pp. 71–88.

Katz, C.L. 2013, 'First person: a mental health mission to post-earthquake El Salvador,' *The Psychiatric Clinics of North America*, vol. 36, no. 3, pp. 309–319.

Maslow, A.H. 1943, 'A theory of human motivation,' *Psychological Review*, vol. 50, no. 4, p. 370.

Satel, S. 2005, *Bread and Shelters, Yes. Psychiatrists, No*. New York Times, March 29. Available: www.nytimes.com/2005/03/29/health/policy/29essa.html?mabReward=relbias:r&adxnnl=1& module=Search&adxnnlx=1418702601-0d8zkSsYJ3zTso8XySCv+w (accessed December 20, 2014).

Schreiber, M. & Gurwich, R. 2006, *Listen, Protect, Connect: Psychological First Aid for Children and Parents*. Available: www.ready.gov/sites/default/files/documents/files/PFA_ Parents.pdf (accessed January 23, 2014).

Southwick, S. & Charney, D. 2012, *Resilience: The Science of Mastering Life's Greatest Challenges*, Cambridge University Press, New York.

Summerfield, D. 2006, 'Survivors of the tsunami: dealing with disaster,' *Psychiatry*, vol. 5, no. 7, pp. 255–256.

Van Moffaert, M. 1998, 'Somatization patterns in Mediterranean migrants,' in S. Okpaku (ed.), *Clinical Methods in Transcultural Psychiatry*, American Psychiatric Press, Inc., Washington, pp. 301–320.

Chapter 10

Placed peoples

After the disaster, hundreds of thousands of people were left displaced from their homes. Flooding was to blame in many areas along the coast, but failures in what was supposed to be reliable infrastructure were to blame elsewhere. Many people had to flee their homes with nothing but what was on their backs and, when it all passed, found there was nothing to return to. Their homes and their communities were either gone or were no longer theirs to inhabit.

It fell to the overwhelmed government to find shelter from the unforgiving elements for its rattled citizens and avert a humanitarian crisis. Schools and stadiums were used at first, becoming converging points for international aid. Temporary housing was erected within weeks so that schools could re-open and people could be offered a modicum of normalcy that was in short supply in the simmering cauldrons of cot-strewn gymnasiums.

Temporary housing was an improvement but was not home. The quarters were tiny and crammed together. In many cases, families were housed far from their communities of origin and far from surviving members of their communities despite having often lived together for centuries. A sense of alienation seemed inescapable in these settlements, whether they were far from town centers or integrated into them. The latter was often no better and sometimes worse, as the evacuees often faced discrimination and resentment from their host communities. Fearing the unknown, many parents refused to let their children even play outside.

Worst of all, there was soon a clear sense that the arrangement was not temporary. Unless the residents were self-sufficient or had welcoming family elsewhere, they were reliant for help on a government that seemed to have no other long term solution other than to leave them there. Thus arose a situation in which those who remained in the settlements were the most helpless and needy and precisely those for whom the government had the least to offer.

It comes as no surprise that this was the situation for many of Sam's beleaguered countrymen following the typhoon that struck their country in the last chapter. But, now re-read the description and realize with likely surprise that it can just as readily be applied to the situation confronting many Japanese people following the 'triple disaster' of March 11, 2011 in which an earthquake spawned a lethal tsunami, which in turn triggered a major nuclear power plant accident in the northeastern Tohoku region of Japan. The radiation leak that led to mass evacuations was due to a failure in 'infrastructure' in the prefecture, or state, of Fukushima (Yamashita & Shigemura 2013). We tend to reflexively think of lower income countries in places like sub-Saharan Africa when we think of the mass displacement of people, but this exercise involving a high income country like Japan has hopefully challenged that misconception.

This chapter seeks to capture the universal anguish of displacement in the lives of people around the globe regardless of the income level of their countries. To do so, we propose reconsidering displacement as *placement* and talking instead about 'placed' peoples. In order to explain what we mean, we will begin with a psychological consideration of house, home, and place. After that we will talk about the utility of a framework of 'placement' by considering the mental health issues across various placed populations—internally displaced people (IDP), refugees, prisoners, and the homeless—and how the global mental health professional can use this concept in practice.

Psychology of house and home

We can look to Freud for some important insights into the human relationship with house and home. He posited that one of the most universal symbols in peoples' dreams was that of the house and suggested that the house in dreams was a stand-in for the human figure. He even went so far as to suggest that dreamt houses with smooth facades were of men whereas those with adornments were female (Freud 1966).

Freud also made a connection between the experience of home and human psychology in his concept of homelessness (Svenaeus 2000; Svenaeus 1999). He is understood to have posited that human beings are born into 'a priori homelessness,' in which many of the activities of their own mind go on beyond their awareness and understanding. To not be entirely 'at home' in one's mind is in fact to be human, as this reflects the unique depth and breadth of the human mind. On the other hand, should the extent of this mystery and disconnect become too profound, it can lead to a level of alienation from oneself that fuels, if not embodies, mental illness. The same can be said of alienation from one's body—the experience of homelessness can rise painfully to the fore when physical illness leads unseen processes beneath the surface of the body to betray the person.

Oft repeated sentiments that 'my body is my home' and 'my body is my temple' reflect the fact that it is not off the mark to say that people fundamentally experience their selves, whether in mind or body, as a house or home. Conversely, one's literal house or home is experienced as an extension of one's self. To have a home is to expand one's footprint on the earth and to thereby expand the scope of one's existence. Homes promise safety, comfort, and affiliation, but they also amount to an existential bid for personal durability, if not immortality. In planting one's flag in the ground, we are expressing a wish to stay above it.

Understanding placement

Having a place of one's own is a seemingly universal way by which people grapple with their mortality and their sense of their finitude. Consider the two ways in which we address this existential challenge. We can believe in our own uniqueness, specialty, and special power; or we can believe that there is something or someone unique and

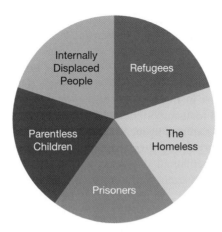

Figure 10.1 The scope of 'placed' populations

special who powerfully looks after us (Yalom 1980). Making a physical place in the world for oneself speaks directly to the former.

Where the individual leans towards a belief in his or her own special power, having a home is the embodiment of such. As an extension of the self, possession of a home reflects expansion of one's size and power. It literally insulates its occupants from the elements and other threats. But, it also communicates to oneself and to others that the individual's frame extends out well beyond himself, rendering them a force they would not otherwise be without it.

Hence, displaced people feel 'placed' and are 'placed' because they were unable to maintain their sense of choice and control over where they live. Losing one's home constitutes a painful reminder of one's smallness and finitude. It delivers a psychological blow that dispels fantasies of control, freedom, and maybe even immortality. And that is why we suggest that displaced people are better considered 'placed' people. 'Displacement' means 'bad' placement, but the more fundamental matter seems to relate to feeling at the mercy of one's world or one's protector. Although a good placement surely helps the matter, a homeowner who loses their home feels less human and more object-like—less the player and more the game-piece. As reflected in Figure 10.1, the global mental health professional should think not just about IDPs and refugees, the two populations that seem to have long been nearly synonymous with global health work, but also prisoners, homeless, and parentless children. IDPs, refugees, prisoners, homeless, and parentless children—all have been placed in places other than their home and all must deal with not only the practicalities but also the emotional implications of this bitter reality. The fifth major group of placed people, parentless children, can overlap with all four of the other populations but also deserves special attention unto itself and has already been covered in Chapter 8.

Internally displaced peoples (IDPs)

The Bosnian civil war of the 1990s exacted an enormous humanitarian toll on that country, including causing the internal displacement of nearly half of its population.

The authors of a study of 1500 Bosnian families found that displacement was associated with a marked sense of powerlessness, loss of a sense of self-sufficiency, and low self-esteem (Carballo et al. 2004). Not surprisingly they also found depressive symptoms and other forms of clinical distress in over 40 percent of the displaced peoples (compared with the already high 19 percent of non-displaced peoples). They made several recommendations for future work with IDPs including inclusion of psychosocial interventions in the broader humanitarian response; keeping together or reuniting families; and focusing on local decision making rather than imposition of policies and activities by external agencies.

Nearly a year after Hurricane Katrina struck the Gulf Coast of the United States, over 2.5 million people remained displaced within the US. A survey of displaced people living in Federal Emergency Management Agency trailers in Louisiana and Mississippi found that 50 percent met criteria for Major Depression, 20 percent reported having suicidal thinking, and 57 percent reported wishing to return to their homes. Overall, the trailer park residents reported that since coming to the trailer park the four biggest problems they faced included lack of privacy, poor security/safety, inadequate finances, and poor transportation. The study authors recommended that these residents not just be regarded as 'evacuees' to be housed but rather as IDPs for whom international standards for rights based care apply (Larrance, Anastario, & Lawry 2007).

Meanwhile, some writers have pointed out that poor African-Americans have faced serial displacement due to a chronic range of social conditions and policies in the United States, causing a range of disruptions, social ills, and health consequences (Fullilove & Wallace 2011). They have suggested that this has created a 'de facto internal refugee population.' It is therefore possible that IDPs can be spawned by non-catastrophic circumstances, although such populations would be harder for the global mental health professional to identify in the absence of a discrete event.

Finally, it is worth remembering that the psychological distress suffered by IDPs relates not just to where they are placed, but also to the trajectory of that placement. Colombia's protracted civil war has produced one of the largest populations of IDPs in the world, a tragedy which research has shown has been beset by severe traumatic exposures. Research has found that the 'trauma signature' of Colombian IDPs encompasses 'very severe' or 'extreme' exposure to eighteen dimensions of hazards, loss, and change (Shultz et al. 2014).

Refugees

Refugees fleeing from a range of countries potentially have about a ten times greater risk of having Post-Traumatic Stress Disorder (PTSD) than the populations of their host countries (Fazel, Wheeler, & Danesh 2005). Although potentially fairing better psychologically than IDPs (Porter & Haslam 2005), refugees uniquely face a range of pre- and post-immigration factors that may bear on their mental health. For example, refugees detained in immigration centers while awaiting asylum determinations in Western countries have high levels of psychiatric distress, including clinical anxiety, PTSD in particular, clinical depression, and suicidality. Evidence also suggests this psychopathology may in part be related to the detention process and detention conditions, including duration (Robjant, Hassan, & Katona 2009). Other post-immigration factors thought to significantly contribute to mental health problems of refugees are institutional or temporary housing, restricted economic opportunity, and ongoing conflict in their home country (Porter & Haslam 2005).

A comprehensive review of 44 studies covering 5766 refugee children displaced to high income countries identified a number of risk and protective factors relevant to their mental health (Fazel et al. 2012). Non-modifiable factors of pre-migration violence exposure and female sex were the most commonly cited mental health risk factors. However, trends were nonetheless found among modifiable factors, as follows: being unaccompanied; exposure to post-migration violence; undergoing multiple post-migration placements; experiencing discrimination; financial stress; or being a child with a single parent or a parent(s) who has experienced violence or has psychiatric problems. Protective factors included having strong parental support and social cohesion, strong support from friends, being in same-ethnicity orphan care, and having a good school experience. As with IDPs, refugees' mental health is affected by both being placed and the experience of how they were placed and of the placement (Fazel et al. 2012).

Prisoners

If ever there were an example of someone being literally 'placed' somewhere without having so chosen, it would of course be prisoners. Whether legally sanctioned or politically motivated, imprisonment by definition divests individuals of much of their freedom as we commonly know it, including the freedom to choose where and how to live. Indeed, inclusion of prisoners among other placed peoples like IDPs and refugees goes beyond mere semantics or theorizing. Like refugees, both the process of their imprisonment (i.e., its duration and legality) and the conditions of their imprisonment surely will affect their mental health.

Others have suggested that localities experiencing high rates of incarceration of community members are effectively being subject to 'forced migration.' The imprisonment of too many members of the community can de-stabilize it and cause disruptions. For example, men are far more likely to be imprisoned than women, leaving the remaining men with far more power (Thomas & Torrone 2006). This may explain why one study has found that statewide rates of teenage pregnancy and sexually transmitted illnesses correlated with rates of incarcerations in North Carolina (Thomas & Torrone 2006).

Mental health professionals probably need not be reminded of the oft discussed problem of prisons becoming de facto psychiatric institutions, but worldwide estimates of prisoner mental health suggest that rates of clinical depression or psychotic disorders are two to four times the rates of the general population (Fazel & Danesh 2002). Substance use disorders, personality disorders (especially anti-social), and PTSD/trauma histories are all also significantly elevated in prisons (Fazel & Baillargeon 2011). And, a 2014 US report found that in 44 of 50 states and the District of Columbia, a state prison or jail contains more seriously mentally ill individuals than does the largest state psychiatric hospital (Torrey et al. 2014).

The global mental health professional should be especially mindful of the needs of prison populations in low resource settings for a number of reasons. First, if mental health resources are low in the general community, they are certainly likely to be even lower to non-existent in their prisons. Most studies of correctional mental health services in high income countries point towards even their being under-resourced (Fazel & Baillargeon 2011). Second, most data available on worldwide prisoner mental health derives from high income countries, leaving prisons in low resource settings as a great unknown (Fazel & Danesh 2002). But, reason suggests the rates must be high, if not higher than Western settings. Third, prisoners in low resource settings potentially suffer significant human rights abuses.

The homeless

The global mental health professional from urban settings in developed countries is likely also familiar with the overlap of mental illness and homelessness (and often incarceration in correctional settings). Of this overlap some advocate for addressing housing first before addressing mental illness, both by increasing access to housing and helping to provide support to maintain the housing (Newman & Goldman 2008). In fact, 'housing first' approaches do seem to lead to more stability and better engagement in psychiatric treatment than 'treatment first' approaches which defer finding a long term housing solution for the mentally ill until they are more stable and skilled. On the other hand, some data suggests that treatment first approaches may actually better help the mentally ill focus on developing higher levels of functioning (including the 'self-actualization' that tops off Maslow's hierarchy), perhaps by frustrating rather than gratifying their basic needs (Henwood et al. 2014). In other words, emphasizing housing first may simply stabilize, even control, the mentally ill without really advancing them socially or professionally.

Ascertaining cause and effect in the consideration of homelessness and mental illness may be theoretically and scientifically challenging, but clinically the housing versus treatment debate is a needless one to have. Mental illness, typically severe mental illness, and homelessness are associated with one another and where one is found the other may not be far behind depending upon a range of modifying factors (i.e., a supportive family). We include the homeless among placed peoples because they, by definition, have lost, or even never had, the ability to exercise usual control over where or how they live.

The homeless are typically associated with high income countries where housing is costlier and family support systems are more fragmented. They should nonetheless fall under the purview of global mental health professionals who are committed, as we defined in the Introduction, to improving access to mental health care 'for all people in all places.' Helping the homeless in one's own community is no less noble than flying off to help Sam's countrymen meet their mental health needs. To overlook them would be to render unseen what we all do see. And, their world on the street may prove to be no less foreign than Sam's country.

Intervening

Guidance on global mental health practice with placed peoples can be distilled from the literature about and experience with the different groups (Table 10.1). First, all placed populations should be able to count on the physical safety of their placements.

Table 10.1 Ways to promote the mental health of placed peoples

1 Ensure their safety
2 Enhance family and social cohesion
3 Promote self-reliance
4 Prioritize a better way of life
5 Provide mental health care

Reducing exposure to violence is crucial as violence of all kinds traumatically proceeds and precipitates placement. To find a safer place when a person has been unwillingly displaced from their home and placed elsewhere is at least to help speak to the existential need to believe someone or something bigger than them has used their power to help them, even amid tragic circumstances. Reducing access to and misuse of alcohol or other substances in resettlement camps like those described in the opening scenario would be an explicit public mental health intervention that would reduce violence of all kinds.

Second, re-establishing, maintaining, or nurturing the cohesiveness and vitality of families and social networks is a central foundation to the health and mental health of all people and especially placed peoples. This is seen in child refugees (Fazel et al. 2012), internally displaced populations (Fullilove & Wallace 2011), and communities plagued by high rates of incarceration (Thomas & Torrone 2006). One study has found that among people displaced by Hurricane Katrina in Mississippi, rates of clinical depression were only elevated compared to non-displaced people in communities found to lack significant social cohesion (Lê et al. 2013). A more difficult question beyond the scope of this book involves approaches to promote familial and social cohesion, although we believe this is relatively unchartered territory at the public health level.

Third, promotion of self-reliance is crucial in placed peoples. This generally involves enhancing economic opportunities. Guidelines for working with IDPs and refugees make the point that the average person uprooted by conflict remains displaced for 17 years, necessitating helping them to begin to help themselves with 'livelihood interventions' such as establishing local camp based micro-economies. On the other hand, in some crisis settings, especially natural disasters, those who remain in temporary housing may be the most vulnerable and needy and thus the most challenging targets for such interventions (Ma et al. 2013). Promotion of self-reliance speaks to both financial and self-esteem needs. We see no reason why this cannot extend to prison communities where local economies, even token ones, can be set up. Prisoners' post-incarceration self-reliance can also be promoted via educational programming and vocational training that are established as part of the rehabilitative missions of prisons. These are all services for which the global mental health practitioner as activist could advocate (see Chapter 4).

Fourth and quite simply at least in theory, implicit in all that has been said is that placed people will be happier and healthier if their placements are better than the places from which they were displaced. Perhaps controversially, we think this should apply to prisoners as well. As helpless and defeated as placement makes people feel, somehow finding themselves in a better place can help to heal the existential wounds gouged into their selves by displacement. Better living conditions, a resilient outlook, religion and spirituality, or such explicit mental health interventions as cognitive-behavioral psychotherapy techniques may abet arriving at the perspective that 'it was for the best after all.' The former is borne out in a study of people relocated from public housing complexes to more scattered public housing integrated into neighborhoods in Atlanta, Georgia, as is typical of recent trends in approaches to public housing (Cooper 2014). Re-location into neighborhoods with less perceived violence or better economic opportunities predicted significant reductions in pre-displacement depression scores.

Lastly, all five groups of placed peoples can be assumed to be reservoirs for high rates of undetected, undiagnosed, or untreated mental illness. In its simplest and most direct form, global mental health efforts with placed populations can involve connecting mental health clinicians with the population of concern to either provide direct care or help train local human resources to provide this care.

Conclusions

Displacement and placement are issues bearing on mental health whether working in high, middle, or low income countries. Specific groups that should be accounted for in global mental health practice are the placed populations—IDPs, refugees, homeless, prisoners, and orphans. The needs of all groups are many and diverse, but the global mental health practitioner can bring to bear their expertise to help them re-orient themselves amid such profound and unsettling change. Here are the essential points for doing so:

✓ Remember that the home holds great psychological meaning in the experience of one's self, an observation that likely crosses cultures (the homesickness of a traveling global mental health practitioner embodies this).
✓ In planning a global mental health program in a community, be sure to ascertain the presence of any of the five populations of placed people and consider them as possible focus of your attention.
✓ If you are invited to assist a particular population of placed peoples, be sure to educate yourself as much as possible about their prior way of life.
✓ The distress that comes from placement can be addressed at the individual, family, or community levels.
✓ Given the multiplicity of needs that arise from placement and as in most areas of global mental health, the global mental health practitioner can maximize their impact on placed peoples by partnering with the range of officials and workers from beyond the fields of health and mental health who are also trying to assist them.

References

Carballo, M., Smajkic, A., Zeric, D., Dzidowska, M., Gebre-Medhin, J., & Van Halem, J. 2004, 'Mental health and coping in a war situation: the case of Bosnia and Herzegovina,' *Journal of Biosocial Science,* vol. 36, no. 4, pp. 463–477.

Cooper, H.L.F. 2014, 'The aftermath of public housing relocations: relationships between changes in local socioeconomic conditions and depressive symptoms in a cohort of adult relocaters,' *Journal of Urban Health,* vol. 91, no. 2, pp. 223; 223–241; 241.

Fazel, M., Wheeler, J. & Danesh, J. 2005, 'Prevalence of serious mental disorder in 7000 refugees resettled in western countries: a systematic review,' *The Lancet,* vol. 365, no. 9467, pp. 1309–1314.

Fazel, M., Reed, R.V., Panter-Brick, C., & Stein, A. 2012, 'Mental health of displaced and refugee children resettled in high-income countries: risk and protective factors,' *The Lancet,* vol. 379, no. 9812, pp. 266–282.

Fazel, S. & Baillargeon, J. 2011, 'The health of prisoners,' *The Lancet,* vol. 377, no. 9769, pp. 956–965.

Fazel, S. & Danesh, J. 2002, 'Serious mental disorder in 23 000 prisoners: a systematic review of 62 surveys,' *The Lancet,* vol. 359, no. 9306, pp. 545–550.

Freud, S. 1966, 'Introductory lectures on psycho-analysis (Parts I and II)' in J. Strachey (ed.), *The Standard Edition of the Complete Psychological Works of Sigmund Freud, Volume XV,* W.W. Norton, New York, pp. 1–240.

Fullilove, M.T. & Wallace, R. 2011, 'Serial forced displacement in American cities, 1916–2010,' *Journal of Urban Health: Bulletin of the New York Academy of Medicine,* vol. 88, no. 3, pp. 381–389.

Henwood, B.F., Derejko, K.S., Couture, J., & Padgett, D.K. 2014, 'Maslow and mental health recovery: a comparative study of homeless programs for adults with serious mental illness,' *Administration and Policy in Mental Health* (Epub ahead of print).

Larrance, R., Anastario, M., & Lawry, L. 2007, 'Health status among internally displaced persons in Louisiana and Mississippi travel trailer parks,' *Annals of Emergency Medicine,* vol. 49, no. 5, pp. 590–601 e12.

Lê, F., Tracy, M., Norris, F.H., & Galea, S. 2013, 'Displacement, county social cohesion, and depression after a large-scale traumatic event,' *Social Psychiatry and Psychiatric Epidemiology,* vol. 48, no. 11, pp. 1729–1741.

Ma, N., Ma, H., He, H., Yu, X., & Caine, E.D. 2013, 'Characteristics of Wenchuan earthquake victims who remained in a government-supported transitional community,' *Asia-Pacific Psychiatry: Official Journal of the Pacific Rim College of Psychiatrists,* vol. 5, no. 2, pp. E73–80.

Newman, S. & Goldman, H. 2008, 'Putting housing first, making housing last: housing policy for persons with severe mental illness,' *The American Journal of Psychiatry,* vol. 165, no. 10, pp. 1242–1248.

Porter, M. & Haslam, N. 2005, 'Predisplacement and postdisplacement factors associated with mental health of refugees and internally displaced persons,' *JAMA: The Journal of the American Medical Association,* vol. 294, no. 5, pp. 602–612.

Robjant, K., Hassan, R., & Katona, C. 2009, 'Mental health implications of detaining asylum seekers: systematic review,' *The British Journal of Psychiatry,* vol. 194, no. 4, pp. 306–312.

Shultz, J.M., Garfin, D.R., Espinel, Z., Araya, R., Oquendo, M.A., Wainberg, M.L., et al. 2014, 'Internally displaced "victims of armed conflict" in Colombia: the trajectory and trauma signature of forced migration,' *Current Psychiatry Reports,* vol. 16, no. 10, p. 475-014-0475-7.

Svenaeus, F. 1999, 'Freud's philosophy of the uncanny,' *Scandinavian Psychoanalytic Review,* vol. 22, no. 2, pp. 239–254.

Svenaeus, F. 2000, 'The body uncanny—further steps towards a phenomenology of illness,' *Medicine, Health Care and Philosophy,* vol. 3, no. 2, pp. 125–137.

Thomas, J.C. & Torrone, E. 2006, 'Incarceration as forced migration: effects on selected community health outcomes,' *American Journal of Public Health,* vol. 96, no. 10, pp. 1762–1765.

Torrey, E.F., Zdanowicz, M., Kennard, A., Lamb, H.R., Eslinger, D.F., Biasotti, M.C., & Fuller, D. 2014, *The Treatment of Persons With Mental Illness In Prisons and Jails: A State Survey*, The Treatment Advocacy Center, Arlington, Virginia.

Yalom, I. 1980, *Existential Psychotherapy*, Basic Books, New York.

Yamashita, J. & Shigemura, J. 2013, 'The Great East Japan Earthquake, tsunami, and Fukushima Daiichi nuclear power plant accident: a triple disaster affecting the mental health of the country,' *The Psychiatric Clinics of North America*, vol. 36, no. 3, pp. 351–370.

Chapter 11

Rural psychiatry

On the left in our photograph we see Molly, an American relief agency volunteer who has been working in the country for the past eight months helping out in the post-disaster effort following the typhoon. Though her work in the country has not focused directly on mental health, she is all too familiar with the territory given that her mother, Silvia, has bipolar disorder.

Silvia lives in a rural community in the State of Montana, surrounded by picturesque mountains and valleys. The nearest community hospital is located 40 miles away from her home. Even though Molly has not lived in Montana for several years, her mother took comfort in knowing she was doing well, living in Seattle, close to her extended family. When Silvia found out that Molly would be working in a far-away developing country doing relief work for an entire year, she worried. For the past months Silvia has been preoccupied with her daughter's safety, and has been losing sleep.

We see Molly on the way to the travel agency, seeking to rebook her flight home. She just received word from an aunt that her mother has been hospitalized again for a 'nervous breakdown.'

Molly's mother faces an all too common scenario in rural America. Living with a chronic mental illness, she struggles to receive appropriate care and does so in a setting where there is little hope for anonymity and a high likelihood of stigmatization. In reality, rural settings in the developed world may present comparable challenges to those encountered in developing countries. In this chapter we will examine the current state of rural mental health care in developed countries and discuss how this might shape the efforts of the mental health professional seeking to work in a rural community in their own country. We will take a look at common systems for rural mental health service delivery, including the prevalent sub-optimal settings as well as effective models of care. A particular example is drawn from a 1970s rural mental health outreach program developed by Duke University in North Carolina. Lessons from rural psychiatry for international psychiatry will also be considered, including the reliance of many US states on telepsychiatry systems. Finally, this chapter also serves as a reminder about the potential extent of mental health needs and practice opportunities in less exotic but still needy places.

The rural setting

Defining rurality

Most people have a fairly clear idea of what a rural setting should look and feel like: farmland, pastures, forests, mountains, small towns, to name a few. Depending on one's own experiences and preferences, these images might conjure up feelings of tranquility and serenity or perhaps isolation, loneliness, and despair. As varied as an individual's response to this setting can be, so are the formal definitions of rurality. Given that population density, landscapes, communal units, and income are all variables with their own scales, it is difficult to draw a defining line between 'urban' and 'rural.' Governmental agencies have for years struggled with finding a universally acceptable measure of rurality, leading to often dichotomous views on whether a particular unit of land should be considered rural or not. The issue is further compounded by the problem of determining what such an entity even consists of: the boundaries of its administrative influence, the way the land is used, or perhaps its economic influence (Cromartie & Bucholtz 2008)?

In the case of health care, defining rurality is equally as ambiguous. It warrants careful thought however because health care delivery depends, to a large extent, on financial structures. The applied definition of rurality will therefore influence fund allocation and research that can drive the expansion and improvement of health care delivery. For example, a township with few medical resources, though fairly close to an urban area, may not be considered underserved due to its proximity to a resource-dense metropolitan area. On closer inspection though, the average travel time to receive care may exceed what is deemed reasonable and acceptable due to poor infrastructure, such as poor roads or public transportation. Depending on how this particular township is captured in a study, it may or may not be labeled as underserved.

Definitions of rurality generally fall into one of three broad categories: spatial, socioeconomic, and sociological. Spatial definitions look at population numbers and density as well as distances to metropolitan areas. Socioeconomic classifications utilize factors such as employment, income, and service delivery characteristics to identify rural settings. Finally, sociological classifications take subjective views of a population into consideration (Nicholson 2008).

Given the multitude of definitions and heterogeneity of research conducted, we will, for the purpose of this chapter, simplify our definition of 'rural' as a setting outside of the fringe of a metropolitan area, where health care access is low. Poor access is in turn defined by both low practitioner density and a high amount of travel time to receive care, particularly specialist care.

It is worth mentioning that a rural setting was the norm for the larger part of human existence on this earth. Only once people started congregating in larger settlements, forming larger towns and cities, was the concept of 'urban' developed. During the age of industrialization migration to the urban centers increased dramatically, leading to our current distribution of the overwhelming majority of people in the developed world living in metropolitan areas (World Bank 2014). This trend has continued to the point where the majority of people *worldwide* are now considered to live in urban areas. Along with this migration came social and demographic changes that have affected rural areas more adversely than urban ones. As Singh and Siahpush

(2002) describe it, a decrease in farming activity and shift towards manufacturing- and service-oriented economies, along with out-migration, may lead to weakening of people's sense of community and social ties.

Unique aspects of rural life

On the one hand, a rural lifestyle can be viewed as idyllic and desirable: open spaces, a peaceful environment, cleaner air and water, a relaxed pace with a lower sense or urgency, higher independence, low rates of criminal and antisocial behavior, as well as a higher reliance on the family and community. While these aspects are all relevant and true, the reality of rural life also comprises statistics showing a higher unemploy-ment/underemployment rate, more elderly people, as well as a higher percentage of poor and uninsured residents (Hart, Larson, & Lishner 2005). Furthermore, rural residents are faced with longer travel times to receive care, fewer practitioners (particularly specialists), and higher medical costs. In certain areas residents can also be faced with a harsh environment due to extreme weather conditions, wildlife, and occupational hazards unique to rural work.

While there is conflicting data on the patterns of prevalence of mental illness in the rural vs. urban settings, the rural environment does evidence a unique set of protective and pathogenic factors in regards to mental health (see Table 11.1).

Physicians practicing in the rural setting have their own set of difficulties. One study conducted in Australia evaluated the positive and negative aspects of working as a physician in a rural environment (Hays et al. 1997). As positive aspects doctors listed the ability to closely interact with a community, to provide a variety of care, to be able to exercise professional autonomy, as well as being able to lead a family-oriented lifestyle. These views generally existed at the beginning of their work experience but were gradually overshadowed by the following issues: a high after-hours workload, a high amount of administrative duties, difficulty obtaining coverage during leave, remoteness from family/friends, and difficulties in obtaining higher education for their children. Needless to say these concerns mirror those of many practitioners in the global setting, as we have learned in our experiences.

Table 11.1 Risk and protective factors for mental illness among rural residents

Protective factors	1 A sense of belonging, to a place and a culture
	2 Closer community ties, with less movement and a high sense of being taken care of
	3 An effective sense of self and how one fits in with the community
	4 A high sense of self-determination in the workplace
	5 Connection with and appreciation of the earth and seasons (Wainer & Chesters 2000)
Risk factors	1 Relative poverty
	2 Relative high rates of alcohol abuse
	3 High prevalence of domestic violence and lack of services to respond
	4 Marginalization of minorities
	5 Increased stigma towards mental illness
	6 Lack of access to mental health care

Epidemiology of rural mental health

The evidence that rates of mental illness are distinctly different in rural vs. urban settings has been inconclusive (Kessler et al. 1994; Nicholson 2008). The question arises, whether any such differences are of particular relevance, when we know that rural communities clearly have less access to care and that their population is under-served (Gamm, Stone, & Pittman 2010; Merwin et al. 2003; Thomas et al. 2009). When comparing the psychiatric morbidity in the urban setting to rural areas, most identified differences disappear when adjusted for confounders such as un-employment, socioeconomic status, ethnicity, educational status, and marital status (Nicholson 2008). This suggests that these factors contribute to mental illness equally in people living in a city or the countryside. Hence, rural communities with higher rates of unemployment, lower socioeconomic status, and low educational states may show higher rates of depression and anxiety (Judd et al. 2002).

There is one exception where prevalence clearly differs: suicide rates tend to be higher in more remote communities, particularly among the young and the elderly (Yip, Callanan, & Yuen 2000; Eberhardt 2001, Singh & Siahpush 2002). This statistic seems to correlate with an increasing sense of social isolation that people living in rural areas may face. Another factor that may contribute to this statistic was identified in a study conducted in North Carolina, which found that elderly people in a rural community tended to have higher expectations of support from family compared to the level they were receiving (Powers & Kivett 1992).

Challenges

The particular characteristics of rural living pose a distinct constellation of challenges that people suffering from mental illness may encounter. We will further discuss the issues of provider shortages below, and will therefore focus our attention on the other factors that may make it difficult for individuals with mental health problems in rural areas.

Remote areas often inherently foster a culture of self-reliance. Harsh environments and limited access to the resources of metropolitan areas require a certain 'do-it-yourself attitude,' which in turn can promote a sense of fortitude towards health problems. Rural inhabitants are less likely to identify themselves as requiring care compared to their urban counterparts despite equal morbidity (Rost et al. 2002; Fox et al. 1999). This phenomenon is also influenced by decreased awareness and educa-tion in regards to mental illness. Rural populations tend to equate mental illness with severe psychiatric disorders, such as schizophrenia, and see depression and anxiety as natural consequences to stressors (Fuller et al. 2000). In one study, rural inhabitants of the US South remained convinced that they did not require help even after screen-ing positive for a mental health problem and receiving educational material (Fox et al. 1999). This tendency alone constitutes an enormous barrier to receiving care (Rost et al. 2002). Efforts to increase access to care therefore need to concentrate on increas-ing the awareness and understanding for seeking help.

Stigma is another significant challenge that people with mental health problems face in rural areas. It is related to their inclination towards stoicism, but is nonetheless an issue in and of itself (Nicholson 2008). Rost et al. found that rural individuals with a history of depression did not feel stigmatized by their community based on their illness, but did perceive labeling associated with seeking treatment (Rost, Smith, & Taylor 1993). Stigma subsequently played a large role in determining whether someone would seek treatment in the rural setting compared to urban areas.

Stigma also plays a greater role in rural communities because of a decreased sense of privacy and confidentiality. Rural communities traditionally show a large flow of information through social gossip networks, which, given a small number of inhabitants, results in a large proportion of the population gaining access to information. The increase in social visibility further compounds the issue that rural inhabitants are more exposed to the consequences of stigma (Aisbett et al. 2007). In some rural areas mistrust of health professionals can be a significant barrier to receiving care, especially in small communities where the provider is tightly integrated and known by everyone.

Rural mental health care systems: United States

It is impossible to quantify and describe psychiatric care for all rural areas of the world, as there are naturally vast regional differences. We will therefore focus on the mental health system in the rural United States, given that a fairly comprehensive amount of research has been conducted there, and because it serves as poignant example of how psychiatric care in a high income country can mimic that of the developing world. Of note, some other regions that have been well researched, and show similar characteristics, are the UK and Australia (Paykel et al. 2000; Gregoire 2002; Aisbett et al. 2007; Griffiths & Christensen 2007).

Mental health care is delivered through various formal and informal routes. Describing a community's access to care via the amount of accessible psychiatrists/ psychologists/psychiatric nurse practitioners/psychiatric beds therefore does not capture other, more informal, types of care. Authors have used the term 'de facto mental health service system' as a way of including all other services (Fox, Merwin, & Blank 1995; Regier et al. 1993). Most Americans in rural settings with a psychiatric illness do not receive appropriate care (Wang et al. 2005).

Formal psychiatric treatment

Most rural counties in the US are considered to be mental health provider shortage areas. The US Health Resources and Services Administration (HRSA) determined that 1 psychiatrist per 10,000 population is an adequate ratio to serve an area's need. Shortage areas are designated to have a ratio equal or higher to 1:20,000, or 1:30,000 depending on the need (Health Resources and Services Administration 2014). In the year 2000 51 percent of all US counties (metropolitan and non-metropolitan) were determined to be Mental Health Professional Shortage Areas (Merwin et al. 2003). When stratified by level of rurality, 76 percent of all counties designated as fully rural (not containing settlements with population >2,500, not adjacent to metro area) were considered mental health shortage areas. These counties had an average of roughly 1 psychiatrist per 100,000 residents (Merwin et al. 2003). While not quite as dismal as in some low income countries, these statistics highlight the striking shortage of providers reminiscent of the global setting (for example Egypt and Iran have similar ratios (World Health Organization 2006)). When including other mental health practitioners in these statistics, the numbers improve somewhat, but remain nonetheless low. The most rural of counties have virtually no child psychiatrists and only 2 psychologists per 10,000 inhabitants. Overall rurality and per capita income are the best predictors of unmet psychiatric need in the United States.

Non-psychiatric resources

Most Americans living in rural areas who receive psychiatric treatment receive it from their primary care practitioner (Fox et al. 1995). While one could argue that at least they are receiving some form of care, one third of primary care patients with psychiatric disorders are unidentified and untreated. And those who do receive treatment are often not referred to specialists. Rural hospitals have few psychiatric beds and most psychiatric patients are treated in scatter beds by non-psychiatric physicians. Emergency rooms also provide psychiatric care when needed and it is estimated that 30–50 percent of emergency admissions in rural hospitals are related to mental illness (Yuen, Gerdes, & Gonzales 1996).

Informal resources represent an important part of psychiatric aid in the rural setting, as in the global setting. Churches and clerics, self-help groups, and volunteer organizations provide help to those in need. There is however little research to provide data on these informal resources. As in the global setting, where psychiatric resources are scarce, human beings tend to seek out friends and family for help.

Effective models of care

Programmatic interventions

Despite the disheartening statistics of rural mental health care, many areas in the US and elsewhere have been able to successfully implement effective rural mental health programs. We will draw an example from a 1970s rural mental health pilot program developed by Duke University in North Carolina and discuss what makes this program effective. We will also take a look at the increasingly important role of telepsychiatry, which has significantly increased access to specialists via videoconferencing technology.

In 1974 the Division of Community Psychiatry at the University of North Carolina published a series of booklets describing a feasibility study conducted from 1967 to 1973 exploring new ways of providing rural mental health care (Hollister 1973). This highly detailed and relevant study carefully delineated the necessary steps to implementing a successful rural mental health program in two rural counties in North Carolina. The program started out small, in order to maximize success and feasibility, and then added features as time and money allowed. Initially a low budget was created, one that would and could be supported by the local community and government. The authors noted that relying heavily on impressive grant monies could lead to overgrown programming that may no longer be supported at the expiration of the grant.

Their approach to the program encompassed the following components:

1   Local control. All University personnel were appointed as county employees in order to foster a sense of community and establish County officials as the owners of the program.

2   Local financial responsibilities. Operations were covered by the County budget.
3   Part-time use of outside specialists. Given difficulties in attracting full-time professionals, part-time specialists were employed. In addition, these specialists were supplemented by gratis professionals such as psychiatric residents and psychology interns.
4   Implementation of local staff. In order to increase acceptance of the program and citizen participation, locals were hired and trained as coordinators, service guides, and secretaries. The coordinators ran day-to-day operations at the mental health center while the service guides performed field visits and helped transport patients to and from the nearest hospital for more intensive care.
5   Using existing resources. Because of a lack of manpower and finances, the psychiatric needs of the local community would have been impossible to meet early on. Strengthening existing support structures not only reduced the workload but also helped with outreach and with providing a referral base.
6   Using a limited clinical program. Due to a lack of resources, the program focused on facilitating severe cases, obtaining help from nearby specialists and then providing local aftercare to prevent relapse. For less severe cases the program utilized the concept of 'helping the helpers.' This included training teachers, nurses, social workers, ministers, and volunteers in relationship skills and mental health. The hope was that these 'helpers' would integrate these skills in their day-to-day work, thereby providing important awareness and preventative interventions.
7   Devoting special effort to consultation, education, prevention, and non-clinical programs.
8   Using citizen participation: while this part of their programming was less fruitful than initially planned, a moderate amount of volunteer help was gained. Volunteers were trained and utilized in various roles, such as clerical staff, transportation services, and even as co-leaders in discussion groups.

The program developed by the University of North Carolina was well thought out and planned, ultimately leading to a significant improvement in the counties' mental health care. It did so by implementing interventions that its creators had evaluated and tested on smaller scales in the years prior to its launch. Interestingly, the very characteristics that made this program successful are still recognized as being essential to developing effective and sustainable programs (US Department of Health and Human Services Health Resources 2011). One of the greatest strengths of the program was its use of local existing resources. By strengthening these resources through training and bridge-building, they were able to reduce their dependence on outside specialists, who are notoriously difficult to attract to remote communities for full-time employment. Partnering with primary care physicians is a vital step, given that most psychiatric patients can be identified in the primary care setting. Furthermore, they were able to create a sense of ownership of the program in the local community, which not only put its success in local stakeholders' hands, but also ensured widespread knowledge of the available resources. Local control, whether financially or through utilization of local staff/volunteers, also ensures that the community's culture, idiosyncrasies, and specific needs are known and addressed. Investing heavily in outreach and education provides additional benefit by de-stigmatizing the act of 'seeing a mental health professional' and can have preventative effects as well. Partnering with the local university and training program provides access to highly educated and highly motivated trainees who can provide essential care at virtually no cost. Interestingly, we have collaborated with several programs in developing countries who have successfully utilized some or all of these strategies to help build up their own mental health program, whether rural or not.

Successful rural health programs in the US tend to focus, at least early on in their inception, on specific goals rather than attempting to 'improve all access to mental health care' (see Table 11.2). For instance, several states identified a specific need for farm workers when this cohort showed an alarmingly high incidence of suicide (Rosmann 2008). Each state created and operated a hotline and website staffed by people with a background in agriculture who received training in mental health. These hotlines provided emergency counseling as well as information about mental health care, legal assistance, financial assistance, and other issues relevant to the farming population (www.agriwellness.org/SSoH.htm).

A program in Alaska, which identified a need for child behavioral health services, created a Youth Leaders Program where volunteer high school students who are natural role models to their peers provide informal counseling to children with behavioral problems (US Department of Health and Human Services Health Resources 2011). The program addresses a dire need through a highly sustainable and affordable framework and has shown a significant decrease in school disciplinary referrals.

In Tennessee, a community health center embeds local behavioral health workers into primary care who can provide screening and brief interventions with patients requiring mild-moderate care. The primary care physicians consult an off-site

Table 11.2 Characteristics of successful rural mental health programs

Relevance to rural	The program is developed specifically for a rural community, or an existing program is adapted in a way that is specific for a rural community.
Impact on rural	The program addresses barriers to behavioral health services in rural communities.
Sustainability	The program ensures sustainability via a reliance on multiple funding sources, and is creative in seeking and obtaining new funding.
Capacity	The program's staff has, or is able to obtain, the qualifications necessary to accomplish the goals of the program.
Documentation of program information	The program has developed marketing materials, effective efforts to communicate with key audiences, and potential funders in their respective communities.
Effectiveness	The program measures and evaluates its effectiveness in order to improve and provide data to funders.
Community engagement	Involving multiple local stakeholders and engaging the community improves outcome and strengthens other aspects of the program.

Source: Adapted from: US Department of Health and Human Services Health Resources 2011

psychiatrist via videoconference who can recommend pharmacological treatment. This last example highlights the growing importance of telepsychiatry in the rural setting (US Department of Health and Human Services Health Resources 2011).

Telepsychiatry

Telepsychiatry refers to the concept of providing psychiatric care from afar using video conferencing technology. Although much more accessible and affordable since the introduction of broadband Internet, telepsychiatry has existed since the late 1950s, when two-way closed-circuit television was first developed (Baer, Elford, & Cukor 1997). High cost and high maintenance of these systems prevented the technology from providing any kind of significant impact and was de facto abandoned. Telepsychiatry has now reemerged as an affordable and accessible tool for providing psychiatric care with a good evidence base (Cuevas et al. 2006; Garcia-Lizana & Munoz-Mayorga 2010; Hilty et al. 2003).

Unlike medical encounters, where physicians often have to be present to do physical exams or perform procedures, psychiatric care can be fairly easily administered without the provider being in the same room as the patient. Both diagnostic assessments as well as psychotherapeutic interventions can be done remotely, and when collaborating with a primary care physician, prescribing of medications is easily accomplished as well.

Several studies dedicated to determining the efficacy of telepsychiatry have shown that diagnosis and follow-up care provided via this technology are equivalent to face-to-face encounters (Cuevas et al. 2006; O'Reilly et al. 2007; Ruskin et al. 2004). This data makes a compelling argument for implementing telepsychiatry in the rural health setting. Generally there are two scenarios how telepsychiatry is practiced, either with the patient at home, using their own personal computer, or using a videoconferencing station set up at a health clinic. Both have advantages and disadvantages. Having a patient participate from their home ensures easy access to care given that many remote areas require significant travel time even to their local rural health clinic. This scenario however requires fairly independent functioning from the patient and is not suited for emergency situations. Telepsychiatry stations in health clinic are more suited to dealing with acute cases, as staff can be on hand to assist and intervene directly. In both cases, the psychiatrist delivering care remotely should be familiar with the local availability of resources and should have a collaborative relationship with local primary care providers. Of note, some programs have utilized telepsychiatry not only to provide direct care, but also to train local staff in behavioral health, thus significantly increasing the impact of this technology.

Practical considerations

We return to Molly's mother, Silvia, and can try to imagine what level of care she is expected to receive at home. For this we shall consider a worst-case and best-case scenario. Most likely she lives in an area without direct mental health services, where a primary care physician is responsible for her care, despite his or her limited knowledge of treating patients with bipolar disorder. Aside from continuing medications that Silvia received while in the hospital, her physician will do little to provide education and psychotherapeutic interventions that can help stabilize her. Silvia's limited insight and lack of family support often lead to medication non-compliance, and although she has strong community ties, she feels uncomfortable sharing that she takes psychiatric medications.

But hopefully Silvia lives in a community with a strong rural mental health program. We could then envision that her community is more enlightened, reducing the stigma she faces and increasing her support system. Perhaps there is a social worker who does home visits to patients with more severe mental illness and who could visit Silvia every few weeks, provide basic counseling, and ensure she is taking her medications. The local medical clinic may even have a telepsychiatry service in place where Silvia can see a psychiatrist that her primary care physician can collaborate with.

As becomes evident, many aspects of rural mental health mirror the challenges that are faced in the global setting. Low resource density, lack of awareness, and stigma contribute to the picture of sub-optimal care that can be provided. This chapter should serve as a reminder that practicing global mental health does not necessarily require a practitioner to travel to exotic or remote places, but that many underserved areas exist right in our own 'backyards,' not far from metropolitan areas. Practitioners seeking to make a difference are as needed in developed countries as in many low income countries as well. Some of the lessons we can glean from rural mental health, which can enhance the global mental health practitioner's knowledge, include the following:

✓ Successful programs are tailored to meet a community's specific need.
✓ Employing and training local human resources enhances credibility, sustain-ability, and cultural appropriateness.
✓ Partnering with existing local helpers improves outcome and lowers cost.
✓ Partnering with a local university or residency training program can provide you with gratis access to highly motivated and trained providers.
✓ Investing in outreach and education helps reduce stigma and has preventative effects.
✓ Telepsychiatry can be an affordable and powerful tool to connect patients and local caretakers with specialists.

References

Aisbett, D., Boyd, C., Francis, K.J., Newnham, K., & Newnham, K. 2007, 'Understanding barriers to mental health service utilization for adolescents in rural Australia,' *Rural and Remote Health,* vol. 7, no. 624, pp. 1–10.

Baer, L., Elford, D.R., & Cukor, P. 1997, 'Telepsychiatry at forty: what have we learned?,' *Harvard Review of Psychiatry,* vol. 5, no. 1, pp. 7–17.

Cromartie, J. & Bucholtz, S. 2008, 'Defining the "rural" in rural America,' *Amber Waves,* vol. 6, no. 3, pp. 28–34.

Cuevas, C.D.L., Arredondo, M.T., Cabrera, M.F., Sulzenbacher, H., & Meise, U. 2006, 'Randomized clinical trial of telepsychiatry through videoconference versus face-to-face conventional psychiatric treatment,' *Telemedicine Journal & e-Health,* vol. 12, no. 3, pp. 341–350.

Eberhardt, M.S. 2001, *Health, United States, 2001: Urban and Rural Health Chartbook*, Department of Health and Human Services, Centers for Disease Control and Prevention, National Center for Health Statistics, Hyattsville, Maryland.

Fox, J.C., Blank, M., Berman, J., & Rovnyak, V.G. 1999, 'Mental disorders and help seeking in a rural impoverished population,' *International Journal of Psychiatry in Medicine*, vol. 29, no. 2, pp. 181–196.

Fox, J., Merwin, E., & Blank, M. 1995, 'De facto mental health services in the rural south,' *Journal of Health Care for the Poor and Underserved*, vol. 6, no. 4, pp. 434–468.

Fuller, J., Edwards, J., Procter, N., & Moss, J. 2000, 'How definition of mental health problems can influence help seeking in rural and remote communities,' *Australian Journal of Rural Health*, vol. 8, no. 3, pp. 148–153.

Gamm, L., Stone, S., & Pittman, S. 2010, 'Mental health and mental disorders—a rural challenge: a literature review,' *Rural Healthy People*, vol. 1, pp. 97–114.

Garcia-Lizana, F. & Munoz-Mayorga, I. 2010, 'What about telepsychiatry? A systematic review,' *Primary Care Companion to the Journal of Clinical Psychiatry*, vol. 12, no. 2, doi:10.4088/PCC.09m00831whi.

Gregoire, A. 2002, 'The mental health of farmers,' *Occupational Medicine*, vol. 52, no. 8, pp. 471–476.

Griffiths, K.M. & Christensen, H. 2007, 'Internet-based mental health programs: a powerful tool in the rural medical kit,' *Australian Journal of Rural Health*, vol. 15, no. 2, pp. 81–87.

Hart, L.G., Larson, E.H., & Lishner, D.M. 2005, 'Rural definitions for health policy and research,' *American Journal of Public Health*, vol. 95, no. 7, pp. 1149–1155.

Hays, R.B., Veitch, P.C., Cheers, B., & Crossland, L. 1997, 'Why doctors leave rural practice,' *Australian Journal of Rural Health*, vol. 5, no. 4, pp. 198–203.

Health Resources and Services Administration 2014, *Medically Underserved Areas/Populations*. Available: www.hrsa.gov/shortage/mua/index.html (accessed January 23, 2014).

Hilty, D.M., Liu, W., Marks, S., & Callahan, E.J. 2003, 'The effectiveness of telepsychiatry: a review,' *Canadian Psychiatric Association Bulletin*, vol. 10, pp. 10–17.

Hollister, W.G. 1973, *Experiences in Rural Mental Health*, Division of Community Psychiatry of the Department of Psychiatry, University of North Carolina, Chapel Hill, North Carolina.

Judd, F.K., Jackson, H.J., Komiti, A., Murray, G., Hodgins, G., & Fraser, C. 2002, 'High prevalence disorders in urban and rural communities,' *Australian and New Zealand Journal of Psychiatry*, vol. 36, no. 1, pp. 104–113.

Kessler, R.C., McGonagle, K.A., Zhao, S., Nelson, C.B., Hughes, M., Eshleman, S., et al. 1994, 'Lifetime and 12-month prevalence of DSM-III-R psychiatric disorders in the United States: results from the National Comorbidity Survey,' *Archives of General Psychiatry*, vol. 51, no. 1, pp. 8–9.

Merwin, E., Hinton, I., Dembling, B., & Stern, S. 2003, 'Shortages of rural mental health professionals,' *Archives of Psychiatric Nursing*, vol. 17, no. 1, pp. 42–51.

Nicholson, L.A. 2008, 'Rural mental health,' *Advances in Psychiatric Treatment*, vol. 14, no. 4, pp. 302–311.

O'Reilly, R., Bishop, J., Maddox, K., Hutchinson, L., Fisman, M., & Takhar, J. 2007, 'Is telepsychiatry equivalent to face-to-face psychiatry? Results from a randomized controlled equivalence trial,' *Psychiatric Services*, vol. 58, no. 6, pp. 836–843.

Paykel, E., Abbott, R., Jenkins, R., Brugha, T., & Meltzer, H. 2000, 'Urban–rural mental health differences in Great Britain: findings from the National Morbidity Survey,' *Psychological Medicine*, vol. 30, no. 2, pp. 269–280.

Powers, E.A. & Kivett, V.R. 1992, 'Kin expectations and kin support among rural older adults,' *Rural Sociology*, vol. 57, no. 2, pp. 194–215.

Regier, D.A., Narrow, W.E., Rae, D.S., Manderscheid, R.W., Locke, B.Z., & Goodwin, F.K. 1993, 'The de facto US mental and addictive disorders service system: epidemiologic catchment area prospective 1-year prevalence rates of disorders and services,' *Archives of General Psychiatry,* vol. 50, no. 2, pp. 85–94.

Rosmann, M.R. 2008, 'Sowing seeds of hope. Providing agricultural communities with crisis services specific to their needs,' *Behavioral Healthcare,* vol. 28, no. 4, pp. 58, 61.

Rost, K., Fortney, J., Fischer, E., & Smith, J. 2002, 'Use, quality, and outcomes of care for mental health: the rural perspective,' *Medical Care Research and Review: MCRR,* vol. 59, no. 3, pp. 231–265; discussion 266–271.

Rost, K., Smith, G.R., & Taylor, J.L. 1993, 'Rural-urban differences in stigma and the use of care for depressive disorders,' *The Journal of Rural Health,* vol. 9, no. 1, pp. 57–62.

Ruskin, P.E., Silver-Aylaian, M., Kling, M.A., Reed, S.A., Bradham, D.D., Hebel, J.R., et al. 2004, 'Treatment outcomes in depression: comparison of remote treatment through telepsychiatry to in-person treatment,' *American Journal of Psychiatry,* vol. 161, no. 8, pp. 1471–1476.

Singh, G.K. & Siahpush, M. 2002, 'Increasing rural-urban gradients in US suicide mortality, 1970-1997,' *American Journal of Public Health,* vol. 92, no. 7, pp. 1161–1167.

Thomas, K., Ellis, A., Konrad, T., Holzer, C., & Morrissey, J. 2009, 'County-level estimates of mental health professional shortage in the United States,' *Psychiatric Services,* vol. 60, no. 10, pp. 1323–1328.

US Department of Health and Human Services Health Resources 2011, *Rural Behavioral Health Programs and Promising Practices*, US Department of Health and Human Services Health Resources and Services Administration Office of Rural Health Policy.

Wainer, J. & Chesters, J. 2000, 'Rural mental health: neither romanticism nor despair,' *Australian Journal of Rural Health,* vol. 8, no. 3, pp. 141–147.

Wang, P.S., Lane, M., Olfson, M., Pincus, H.A., Wells, K.B., & Kessler, R.C. 2005, 'Twelve-month use of mental health services in the United States: results from the National Comorbidity Survey Replication,' *Archives of General Psychiatry,* vol. 62, no. 6, pp. 629–640.

World Bank 2014, *Data | The World Bank*. Available: http://data.worldbank.org/ (accessed January 23, 2014).

World Health Organization 2006, *WHO–AIMS Report on Mental Health System in Nepal*, World Health Organisation & Ministry of Health and Population, Nepal. Available: www.who.int/mental_health/evidence/nepal_who_aims_report.pdf (accessed November 1, 2007).

Yip, P.S., Callanan, C., & Yuen, H.P. 2000, 'Urban/rural and gender differentials in suicide rates: east and west,' *Journal of Affective Disorders,* vol. 57, no. 1, pp. 99–106.

Yuen, E.J., Gerdes, J.L., & Gonzales, J.J. 1996, 'Patterns of rural mental health care: an exploratory study,' *General Hospital Psychiatry,* vol. 18, no. 1, pp. 14–21.

Part 4

Special issues

Chapter 12

Psychiatric abuses and neglect

During the dictatorship that fomented the civil war, George the pharmacist's father was a vocal member of the opposition. A lawyer known for advocating for clients regardless of ability to pay, he inevitably became an important voice of the people during the period of oppression. However, his preeminence also placed him squarely in the crosshairs of the government, which eventually labeled him a 'psychotic menace.' A government psychiatrist committed him to the country's psychiatric hospital, where George's father was treated with antipsychotic medications and confined to a locked ward. Heavily sedated throughout, he fell down a small flight of stairs going to the latrine and suffered a severe head injury for which he received no medical attention. When George's father was finally released during the civil war, he could not return to work as an attorney due to sequelae of what was eventually diagnosed as a traumatic brain injury. George's eldest brother became the breadwinner for all of them.

Good will fuels the field of global mental health, and its ambitions can seem beyond reproach. For its practitioners, its most evident failing resides in the disparity between the loftiness of its ambitions and the reality of its accomplishments. However, others can and sometimes do differ. It is the very intentions of the practitioner that are subject to anything from skepticism to fear. As with George's father, recent history confirms that psychiatry can be misused within countries for political ends (Bonnie 1990; Munro 2000). Psychiatric abuses also include inappropriate experimentation, including those done with suspected spies in the name of state security (Gunn 2006). Questions have also been raised about the hegemonic nature of the field when practitioners travel from one country to another bearing its ostensible riches. Finally, beyond its commissions, the field of mental health can and has also been criticized for its omissions and what it has neglected. Believing that an 'ounce of prevention is worth a pound of cure' we here examine why host communities may greet the global mental health practitioner with fear or mistrust.

Political use of psychiatry

At least three factors conspire in predisposing psychiatry to being co-opted for state suppression of political dissidents like George's father (Alexander 1997). First, the stigmatizing nature of mental illness across so many cultures (see Chapter 13) makes it an easily deployed tool for casting people to the margins of society by labeling them as mentally ill. Second, ongoing scientific and social debate as to what constitutes mental illness lends malleability to this label. Third, in general, there are less civil protections and procedures surrounding commitment of designated psychiatric patients as compared to criminal imprisonment.

The political misuse of psychiatry has been well documented in a number of authoritarian countries, most notably the former Soviet Union and China. In the former Soviet Union, allegations of psychiatric oppression of political dissidents emerged in the 1970s and led to condemnation by the World Psychiatric Association (WPA) and eventual resignation of the Soviet All-Union Society for Neuropathologists and Psychiatrists from the WPA before it could be expelled. A glasnost inspired investigative delegation of US psychiatrists traveled to the Soviet Union in 1989, and its report led to eventual reforms (Bonnie 1990).

However, importantly for global mental health professionals, it has been suggested that it is not clear from the delegation's report and what is otherwise known about the Soviet practice of psychiatry at the time whether the overuse of inpatient psychiatric commitment in that era was entirely the result of intentional misdiagnosis of dissidents. There were in fact many cases where dissidents did fit Soviet criteria for psychiatric diagnoses such as mild or moderate schizophrenia that would not have met criteria according to Western diagnostic systems (Bonnie 2002, 1990). Taken in cross-cultural terms, this already complex debate about the respective roles of 'evil doctors' or 'bad medicine' can be expanded to include the possibility of 'different' medicine. Similar considerations have been raised about South Africa, where oppressive apartheid era thinking inevitably influenced the psychological framework under which post-apartheid South Africans have received mental health care, with or without malevolent intentions on the part of the mental health establishment (Mkhize 1994).

Communist China is also thought to have adopted Soviet style coercive psychiatry (Bonnie 2002). In fact, an exhaustive investigation suggests that a small community of 'forensic psychiatrists' in Communist China took such measures to a greater extreme (Munro 2000). The Cultural Revolution in particular distinguished between 'genuine' political offenders and so-called 'political lunatics,' the practical effect of which was still to deprive each of their freedom. Both would be deemed criminals, but where the former were criminally imprisoned, the latter were placed in police-run psychiatric custody. In the 1980s, China established a network of police-run facilities known as Ankang to handle mentally ill offenders (Appelbaum 2001). It is also believed that China's crackdown on the Falan Gong religious sect has involved psychiatric detention, albeit in general psychiatric hospitals and amid ongoing debate even in the West as to the psychiatric status of Falan Gong followers (Appelbaum 2001; Munro 2000; Bonnie 2002).

After decades of failed attempts, China attained what some have called a 'high water mark' in 2013 in passing a new mental health law meant to reform their psychiatric system and bring it more in line with the systems in high income countries (Phillips et al. 2013). Its provisions include an emphasis on voluntary psychiatric treatment and the prohibition of political uses of psychiatric care. Nonetheless, human rights activists have questioned whether the law is stringent enough to truly eliminate politically motivated psychiatric detention, including release of previously detained dissidents (Human Rights Watch 2013).

Beyond the use of psychiatry for political repression, there are also abundant other examples of the misuse of psychiatry, including for torture and even military purposes (Lopez-Munoz, et al. 2007). Note the prescription of stimulants to Japanese 'kamikaze pilots' and to Allied troops in World War II to promote not only alertness but also combativeness. The latter highlights that non-clinical and potentially anti-humanitarian uses of psychiatry are not limited to totalitarian regimes, as does a legacy of blatantly unethical psychiatric experimentation with such techniques as 'brain-washing' by the US Central Intelligence Agency (Lopez-Munoz et al. 2007).

Eugenics

The euthanizing of populations deemed deviant, undesirable, or burdensome, including the mentally ill, constituted a major policy of the Nazi regime in Germany, even if it were never written into law (Emerson Vermaat 2002). Justified if not rationalized as 'mercy killings,' these often served as opportunities to experiment with killing methods later used in concentration camps. Across the six 'Operation T-4' euthanasia centers around Nazi Germany, psychiatrists were for the first time actively killing psychiatric patients, including the gassing or cremation of over 10,000 psychiatric patients at the Hadamar Psychiatric Institute during the first nine months of 1941 alone (Strous 2006).

However, the monstrosity of these murders and their unequivocal immorality should not necessarily offer us comfort that they and the like are beyond the pale in other societies, including democratic ones. Eugenic sterilization laws were passed in the United States before even Nazi Germany did so in 1933, and even while the Nazis were actively killing psychiatric patients, American physicians debated the use of euthanasia in psychiatry in 1942 issues of the flagship journal of the American Psychiatric Association (Joseph 2005). Although taken to a virulent and violent extreme in Germany, early 20th century eugenics movements in England and the US were sources for Nazi eugenic policies (Pilgrim 2008). In the early 2000s the Netherlands even legalized euthanasia, albeit admittedly with strict guidelines (Emerson Vermaat 2002).

Writers on the history of eugenics repeatedly suggest that modern Western psychiatry retains eugenic strains even if not eugenic practice (Pilgrim 2008; Emerson Vermaat 2002). They point specifically to attempts to rate cognitive abilities and to the modern bias towards the potential reductionism of biological psychiatry over the broad-based 'biopsychosocial model' of psychiatry (Pilgrim 2008). It is not clear to us that this analogy holds up at all, especially since biological psychiatry seeks to address mental illness through biological interventions rather than taking genetics to be inalterable fate. But, there is at least a historical cautionary tale here in the fact that prior to the rise of the Nazis, German psychiatry was held in high international esteem internationally for many things, including its ethics (Birley 2000). That German psychiatry was seen as a model for emulation by psychiatrists and other mental health professionals around the world prior to its ethical nosedive during the Nazi era (possibly due to the post World War I economic pressures) should humble any global mental health professional working to bring the Western psychiatric model to those who lack it.

Hegemony

This then relates to another charge against psychiatry and in the case specifically against global mental health, namely that it is imperialistic (Mills 2014; Summerfield 2008). This anti-global mental health movement rests on several premises, namely that Western psychiatry (1) engages in diagnostic practices that rest on shaky scientific grounds; (2) mistakenly assumes its diagnostic scheme has cross-cultural relevance; and (3) de-emphasizes social and economic determinants of mental health and overemphasizes biological ones. Of the countless people around the world living in intractable poverty, these writers glibly ask various versions of, 'Would antidepressants and Western talk therapy improve their lot?' (Summerfield 2013). Their critique eventually comes around to the contention that the Western pharmaceutical industry lies behind the field of global mental health, seeking to open up new markets in which to peddle their snake oils. In this view, global mental health practitioners are modern day colonizers.

We call attention to this school of thought in part out of fairness to opposing views, even one whose conclusions are so in opposition to the ideas of this book as to question its legitimacy. We also do so because while their conclusions about the imperialistic and capitalistic nature of global mental health professionals seem entirely wrong, their premises are not entirely off base. Western psychiatry diagnoses are potentially problematic and oft debated; their cross-cultural relevance should always be examined; and no mental health professional who questions the role of the environment, including economic, social, and political circumstances in which people find themselves, in how people feel, think, and act is worthy of their title (see Chapter 4 on socioeconomic conditions). But, anyone who has ever tried to help improve the availability of psychotropic drug supplies in low resource settings and finds that the best they can do is collect a hodgepodge of pharmaceutical samples in a knapsack knows that the pharmaceutical industry's indifferent rather than rapacious attitude towards global mental heath is our challenge.

Neglect

So far we have discussed all of the potential ways in which psychiatry can and has been misused. We round out this discussion by highlighting what is surely a much bigger practical problem even if less of an ethical one—how much psychiatry is 'under-used.' In a very real sense this is the underlying premise of this book— that there are too many cases of undiagnosed and untreated mental illness (see Chapter 1 on epidemiology) and too few resources (see Chapters 2 and 3 on the shortfall of resources available to remedy this matter). But, we specifically want to call attention to how much of an issue the neglect of mental illness remains even in high income countries in order to underscore the global nature of the problem.

We specifically think of the United States, where the de-institutionalization movement of the 1970s sought to correct horrific abuses in psychiatric facilities by closing state mental health hospitals (Greenblatt and Glazier 1975). Willbrook Hospital in Staten Island, New York was perhaps the most famous case of overcrowded and dangerous hospitals, having been labeled a 'snake pit' by then Senator Robert F.

Kennedy and a 'concentration camp' for its developmentally and intellectually delayed patients by one of its own psychiatrists (Keitzman & Jerian 2013). The closing of state psychiatric hospitals proved a solution to the neglectful, disempowering custodial care that had become synonymous with institutional care and was an important turning point in the patient advocacy and community psychiatry movements (Watson & Wright 2014). For global mental health professionals who have encountered 'snake pits' in many countries around the world, psychiatric hospitals in places like the United States were not any different not too long ago.

On the other hand, the well-intentioned de-institutionalization movements in countries like the United States have never fully lived up to their promise of investing in community psychiatric resources. Described 'as the most well-meaning but poorly planned medical-social policy of twentieth-century America,' de-institutionalization left a different and more insidious form of neglect in its wake (Torrey et al. 2014). Jails and prisons have become the de facto institution in which many mentally ill patients in the United States have come to reside given the distressingly high rates of mental illness among criminal offenders (perhaps as high as nearly one third of female inmates) (Steadman et al. 2009). As discussed in Chapter 10 and perhaps for different historical reasons as most countries lack a public mental health system to close in the first place, this is a worldwide issue as well (Fazel & Danesh 2002). Unlike Soviet era 'psychiatrization' of otherwise mentally healthy political opposition in lieu of their criminalization, we might say we now encounter criminalization of mentally ill people in lieu of their psychiatrization.

Protections

In addressing the abuse and neglect of psychiatry around the world while themselves avoiding becoming a vehicle for the misuse of psychiatry, global mental health professionals have ethical conventions and codes at their disposal to guide how they, their colleagues, and society at large treat sufferers of mental illness.

The UN Convention on the Rights of Persons with Disabilities entered into force in 2008 (United Nations 2008). Many of its articles pertain to the mentally ill or those labeled as such, including Article 5, which guarantees equal treatment free of discrimination; Article 12, which articulates that people with disabilities deserve equal recognition before the law; Article 15, which declares that they should have freedom from torture or cruel or unusual punishment; and Articles 27–30, which collectively address the rights of people with disabilities to be full participants in the work, political, and social dimensions of society. Table 12.1 lists other key international agreements that relate to mental health, including some that are global and others that are regional in scope. The WHO QualityRights Tool Kit for improving quality and human rights in mental health and social care facilities provides an excellent review of other human right instruments relevant to mental health and lays out a format for assessing and reporting human rights violations in these facilities (WHO 2012).

With only some variation, professional codes of conduct also address matters relevant to global mental health practice. Codes exist for the many health and public health fields central to the practice of global mental health, including psychiatry (American Psychiatric Association 2013), psychology (American Psychological

Table 12.1 Major international declarations, conventions, and codes of relevance to the ethical treatment of persons with mental illness

Universal Declaration of Human Rights	Everyone has the right to a standard of living adequate for the health and wellbeing of himself and of his family, including food, clothing, housing and medical care and necessary social services, and the right to security in the event of unemployment, sickness, disability, widowhood, old age or other lack of livelihood in circumstances beyond his control. (www.un.org/rights/50/decla.htm)
Convention on the Rights of Persons with Disabilities	Persons with disabilities include those who have long-term physical, mental, intellectual or sensory impairments which in interaction with various barriers may hinder their full and effective participation in society on an equal basis with others. (www.un.org/disabilities/convention/conventionfull.shtml)
International Covenant on Economic, Social, and Cultural Rights	The States Parties to the present Covenant recognize the right of everyone to the enjoyment of the highest attainable standard of physical and mental health. (www.ohchr.org/EN/ProfessionalInterest/Pages/cescr.aspx)
International Covenant on Civil and Political Rights	No one shall be subjected to torture or to cruel, inhuman or degrading treatment or punishment. In particular, no one shall be subjected without his free consent to medical or scientific experimentation. (www.ohchr.org/en/professionalinterest/pages/ccpr.aspx)
Convention against Torture and Other Cruel, Inhuman, or Degrading Treatment or Punishment	For the purposes of this Convention, the term 'torture' means any act by which severe pain or suffering, whether physical or mental, is intentionally inflicted on a person for such purposes as obtaining from him or a third person information or a confession, punishing him for an act he or a third person has committed or is suspected of having committed, or intimidating or coercing him or a third person, or for any reason based on discrimination of any kind, when such pain or suffering is inflicted by or at the instigation of or with the consent or acquiescence of a public official or other person acting in an official capacity. (www.ohchr.org/EN/ProfessionalInterest/Pages/CAT.aspx)
African Charter on Human and Peoples' Rights	Every individual shall have the right to enjoy the best attainable state of physical and mental health. (www.achpr.org/instruments/achpr/)
American Convention on Human Rights	Every person has the right to have his physical, mental, and moral integrity respected. No one shall be subjected to torture or to cruel, inhuman, or degrading punishment or treatment. All persons deprived of their liberty shall be treated with respect for the inherent dignity of the human person. (www.oas.org/dil/treaties_B-32_American_Convention_on_Human_Rights.htm)
Inter-American Convention on the Elimination of All Forms of Discrimination against Persons with Disabilities	To achieve the objectives of this Convention, the states parties undertake to collaborate effectively in ... the development of means and resources designed to facilitate or promote the independence, self-sufficiency, and total integration into society of persons with disabilities, under conditions of equality. (www.oas.org/juridico/english/treaties/a-65.html)

Table 12.1 Continued

European Convention for the Protection of Human Rights and Fundamental Freedom	No one shall be deprived of his liberty save in the following cases and in accordance with a procedure prescribed by law: the lawful detention of persons for the prevention of the spreading of infectious diseases, of persons of unsound mind, alcoholics or drug addicts or vagrants. (http://conventions.coe.int/treaty/en/treaties/html/005.htm)
World Medical Association Declaration of Helsinki	Ethical principles for medical research involving human subjects. (www.wma.net/en/30publications/10policies/b3/)
World Psychiatric Association Madrid Declaration	Ethical standards for all aspects of psychiatric practice. (www.wpanet.org/detail.php?section_id=5&content_id=48)

Association 2010), public health (Public Health Leadership Society 2002), psychiatric nursing (International Society of Psychiatric Mental Health Nurses 2006), and social work (National Association of Social Work 2008).

Conclusion

The global mental health practitioner must both address the abuse and neglect of psychiatry and avoid becoming perpetrators of these violations. We believe the chances of the latter are far less than the challenges posed by the former. Nonetheless, where mental health professionals are missing from a community's history or, worse, part of a dark history, the global mental health practitioner will be challenged to address misperceptions about their intentions and their influence.

In this regard, we suggest you keep the following points in mind:

✓ Thinking of the country/community as your 'patient,' consider its own 'past psychiatric history,' specifically gauging its historical experience with psychiatric abuses or neglect.
✓ Where abuses have transpired, carefully weigh how much they were born of malevolence versus incompetence.
✓ Familiarize yourself with the UN Convention on the Rights of Persons with Disabilities and other international conventions and then periodically re-familiarize yourself with them, especially those specific to the given region in which you are working.
✓ Review your profession's ethical code before any global mental health mission, using its relevant principles to orient how you plan it, execute it, and assess it.
✓ Consider the UN Convention and your ethical code of conduct your sword and your shield, fortifying your efforts and safeguarding your ethics.

References

Alexander, G. 1997, 'International human rights protection against psychiatric political abuses,' *Santa Clara Law Review*, vol. 37, pp. 387–426.

American Psychological Association 2010, *Ethical Principles of Psychologists and Code of Conduct*, American Psychological Association, Washington, D.C.

American Psychiatric Association 2013, *The Principles of Medical Ethics with Annotations Especially Applicable to Psychiatry*. American Psychiatric Association, Arlington, Virginia.

Appelbaum, P.S. 2001, 'Law & psychiatry: abuses of law and psychiatry in China,' *Psychiatric Services*, vol. 52, no. 10, pp. 1297–1298.

Birley, J.L. 2000, 'Political abuse of psychiatry,' *Acta Psychiatrica Scandinavia*, vol. 399, pp. 13–15.

Bonnie, R.J. 1990, 'Soviet psychiatry and human rights: reflections on the report of the U.S. Delegation,' *Law, Medicine & Health Care: A Publication of the American Society of Law & Medicine*, vol. 18, no. 1–2, pp. 123–131.

Bonnie, R.J. 2002, 'Political abuse of psychiatry in the Soviet Union and in China: complexities and controversies,' *The Journal of the American Academy of Psychiatry and the Law*, vol. 30, no. 1, pp. 136–144.

Emerson Vermaat, J.A. 2002, '"Euthanasia" in the Third Reich: lessons for today?' *Ethics & Medicine*, vol. 18, no. 1, pp. 21–32.

Fazel, S. & Danesh, J. 2002, 'Serious mental disorder in 23 000 prisoners: a systematic review of 62 surveys,' *The Lancet*, vol. 359, no. 9306, pp. 545–550.

Greenblatt, M. & Glazier, E. 1975, 'The phasing out of mental hospitals in the United States,' *American Journal of Psychiatry*, vol. 132, pp. 1135–1140.

Gunn, J. 2006, 'Abuse of psychiatry,' *Criminal Behaviour and Mental Health*, vol. 16, pp. 77–86.

Human Rights Watch 2013, *China: End Arbitrary Detention in Mental Health Faciities*. Available: www.hrw.org/news/2013/05/03/china-end-arbitrary-detention-mental-health-institutions (accessed July 28, 2014).

International Society of Psychiatric Mental Health Nurses 2006, *Psychiatric Mental Health Nursing Scope & Standards, Draft Revision 2006*. Available: www.ispn-psych.org/docs/standards/scope-standards-draft.pdf (accessed December 16, 2014).

Joseph, J. 2005, 'The 1942 "euthanasia" debate in the *American Journal of Psychiatry*,' *History of Psychiatry*, vol. 16, no. 2, pp. 171–179.

Keitzman, P.R. & Jerian, K.E. 2013, 'Willowbrook: precedent or promise? Modification of consent decrees following the Second Circuit's 1983 decision,' in *NYSARC v. Carey*, pp. 587–602. Available: http://heinonline.org/HOL/LandingPage?handle=hein.journals/aglr6&div=27&id=&page= (accessed December 15, 2014).

Lopez-Munoz, F., Alamo, C., Dudley, M., Rubio, G., Garcia-Garcia, P., Molina, J.D. & Okasha, A. 2007, 'Psychiatry and political-institutional abuse from the historical perspective: the ethical lessons of the Nuremberg Trial on their 60th anniversary,' *Progress in Neuro-psychopharmacology & Biological Psychiatry*, vol. 31, no. 4, pp. 791–806.

Mills, C. 2014, *Decolonizing Global Mental Health: The Psychiatrization of the Majority World*, Routledge, London.

Mkhize, H. 1994, 'Violent oppression: implications for mental health policy in South Africa,' *Medicine and Law*, vol. 13, pp. 193–203.

Munro, R. 2000, 'Judicial psychiatry in China and its political abuses,' *Columbia Journal of Asian Law*, vol. 14, p. 1.

National Association of Social Work 2008, *Code of Ethics of the National Association of Social Work*, 2008 draft revision. Available: www.socialworkers.org/pubs/code/code.asp (accessed December 16, 2014).

Phillips, M.R., Chen, H., Diesfeld, K., Xie, B., Cheng, H.G., Mellsop, G., & Liu, X. 2013, 'China's new mental health law: reframing involuntary treatment,' *The American Journal of Psychiatry,* vol. 170, no. 6, pp. 588–591.

Pilgrim, D. 2008, 'The eugenic legacy in psychology and psychiatry,' *The International Journal of Social Psychiatry,* vol. 54, no. 3, pp. 272–284.

Public Health Public Health Leadership Society 2002, *Principles of the Ethical Practice of Public Health,* Version 2.2. Available: www.apha.org/~/media/files/pdf/about/ethics_brochure.ashx (accessed December 16, 2014).

Steadman, H., Osher, F., Robbins, P.C., Case, B., & Samuels, S. 2009, 'Prevalence of serious mental illness among jail inmates,' *Psychiatric Services,* vol. 60, no. 6, pp. 761–765.

Strous, R.D. 2006, 'Nazi euthanasia of the mentally ill at Hadamar,' *American Journal of Psychiatry,* vol. 163, no. 1, p. 27.

Summerfield, D. 2008, 'How scientifically valid is the knowledge base of global mental health?,' *BMJ (Clinical research edn.),* vol. 336, no. 7651, pp. 992–994.

Summerfield, D. 2013, '"Global mental health" is an oxymoron and medical imperialism,' *British Medical Journal,* vol. 346, p. f3509.

Torrey, E.F., Zdanowicz, M., Kennard, A., Lamb, H.R., Eslinger, D.F., Biasotti, M.C., & Fuller, D. 2014, *The Treatment of Persons With Mental Illness In Prisons and Jails: A State Survey,* The Treatment Advocacy Center, Arlington, Virginia. Available: http://tacreports.org/treatment-behind-bars (accessed December 15, 2014).

United Nations 2008, *Convention on the Rights of Persons with Disabilities.* May 3, 2008 last update. Available: www.un.org/disabilities/default.asp?navid=15&pid=150 (accessed August 3, 2014).

Watson, D.P. and Wright, E.R. 2014, 'Treatment of mental illness in the United States,' in W. Cockerham, R. Dingwall, & S. Quah (eds.), *The Wiley-Blackwell Encyclopedia of Health, Illness, Behavior, and Society,* John Wiley & Sons, Oxford, pp. 1623–1626.

World Health Organization 2012, *WHO QualityRights Tool Kit to Assess and Improve Quality and Human Rights in Mental Health and Social Care Facilities,* Geneva, World Health Organization. Available: www.who.int/mental_health/publications/QualityRights_toolkit/en/ (accessed December 16, 2014).

Chapter 13

Stigma

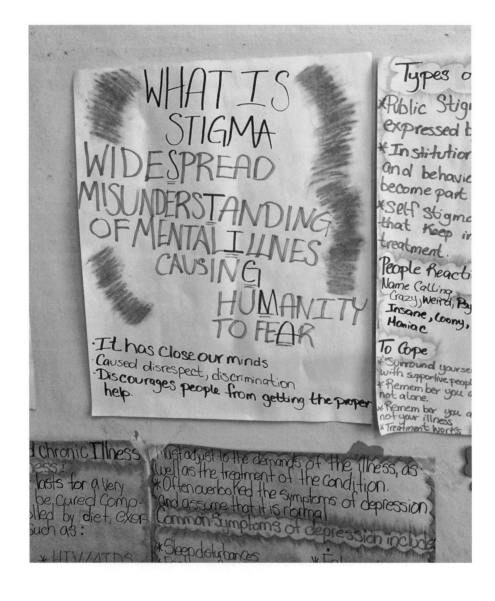

We discovered this sign about stigma in the waiting room of a public mental health clinic in Belize. It was written by nursing students rotating through the clinic who astutely zeroed in on how much of a role stigma played in the lives of the psychiatric patients they were meeting. It is hard to imagine finding a comparable poster voicing awareness of stigma, let alone of the existence of mental illness, in Sam's country as we have come to know it. Indeed, this was a unique find for most any place in the world.

The students' acronym was a sincere approach to somehow making sense of stigma—*wideSpread misundersTanding of mental Illness causinG huManity to feAr*. In this chapter, we will make our own attempt to do the same. We will define stigma and the sub-concept of self-stigma, elaborate on stigma's relationship to mental health, and discuss the how and, ultimately, the why of intervening to address stigma.

Defining stigma

Stigma arises when someone becomes equated with a socially unacceptable physical, characterological, or social trait of theirs, leaving their overall identity 'discredited' and them cut off from a disapproving society if not from their own disapproving selves (Goffman 1963). Embodying 'social-status loss and discrimination triggered by negative stereotypes that have become linked in a particular society,' it has been described as a 'second disease' that can be both cause and effect of mental illness (Krajewski et al. 2013). Stigmatization takes place on three levels: institutional (structural stigma); interpersonal (social stigma); and individual (self-stigma) (Livingston & Boyd 2010).

The World Health Organization has helpfully distinguished between three related concepts. Stigma reflects an *attitude* that involves making unfair moral judgments about others. Discrimination involves unfair *treatment* of people, whether intentional or not. Finally, *social exclusion* involves people's being unable to participate in society as they would like and consequently suffering a loss of otherwise available opportunities. Social exclusion results from stigma and discrimination (WHO 2008).

Self-stigma

Self-stigma or internalized stigma refers to the internalization of public stigma. In the psychiatric realm, internalization of stigma occurs when a person cognitively or emotionally absorbs stigmatizing assumptions and stereotypes about mental illness and comes to believe and apply these to themselves (Drapalski et al. 2013). Self-stigma could even arise whether or not they have mental illness, having more to do with how much they identify with the mentally ill. Nonetheless, rates of self-stigma are high in mentally ill populations, with moderate to severe self-stigma found in 35 percent of one sample of African-American psychiatric outpatients with mood or psychotic disorders (Drapalski et al. 2013).

Self-stigma has pervasively pernicious effects on people. The self-stigmatized individual feels de-valued and marginalized. Their sense of there being a meaning in their lives can be especially affected by self-stigma, especially when they are highly insightful about their mental illness (Ehrlich-Ben Or et al. 2013). As such, it can have significant effects on most major dimensions of people's lives, spawning drop in income, unemployment, less socializing, and even reduced adherence to psychiatric treatment, whether pharmacologic or otherwise (Boyd et al. 2014). At the same time, it appears to be a phenomenon that crosses cultures in fairly universal ways. Indeed, the Internalized Stigma of Mental Illness Scale has been translated into and studied in 55 different languages (Boyd et al. 2014).

Self-stigma itself can be broken down into a subset of interrelated events (Corrigan et al. 2006). First, the individual must become aware of public stigma around mental illness. Second, they adopt and apply it to people with mental illness (stereotype agreement). Third, they apply it to themselves. And, subsequently, their self-esteem and/or self-efficacy suffer.

Stigma and mental health diagnoses

Stigma has been associated with a range of psychiatric disorders. Among sufferers of schizophrenia spectrum disorders, a review of various studies found an overall rate of experienced stigma of over 55 percent (Gerlinger et al. 2013). Structural stigma was overall experienced 26.6 percent of the time and an interpersonal impact of stigma was found in over 49 percent of subjects across studies. Over a third of subjects experienced diminished personal and occupational opportunities.

Among people with mood and/or anxiety disorders, one study found stigma reported at a rate of 22.1 percent in developing countries and 11.7 percent in developed countries (Alonso et al. 2008). As mentioned in Chapter 1, stigma has been found to confront clinical depression less than schizophrenia across a range of countries but still poses an issue for both conditions (Pescosolido et al. 2013). And, there appears to be what investigators have called a 'backbone' of stigmatizing attitudes common to both— reluctance to have sufferers of either teach or care for a child or to be an in-law and belief that both groups are violent or unpredictable (Pescosolido et al. 2013).

Both perceptions of public stigma and self-stigma likely contribute to under-utilization of mental health services by the otherwise high risk military population (Vogt 2011). For example, among American war veterans from the Iraqi and Afghanistan wars, mental health stigma has posed an obstacle to seeking care for Post-Traumatic Stress Disorder, Major Depression, or Alcohol Use Disorder (Pietrzak et al. 2009).

Stigma across countries and communities

As in the just referenced study about stigma about mood and anxiety disorders, we typically associate mental health stigma with low and middle income countries or non-Western or rural settings. In further support of this common wisdom, a comparison of medical students from Ghana and Australia found that the Ghanaian students held significantly more stigmatizing attitudes towards mental health issues and Australian more positive attitudes (Lyons et al. 2014). Nonetheless, stigma was still an issue in both groups. In fact, rates of mental health stigma appear to be on the rise in many countries, including high income countries (Rusch, Angermeyer, & Corrigan 2005).

Japan represents a high income country where issues of mental health stigma abound (Ando et al. 2013). On the whole, prevailing attitudes in Japan doubt the possibility of recovering from mental illness, attributing such problems to personal weakness and begetting much social distancing of people known to be mentally ill. Possible explanations for this constellation of highly stigmatized thinking and behaviors include Japanese psychiatry's emphasis on institutionalization over community care and cultural emphasis on conformity (Ando et al. 2013).

Likely related is a separate finding that 'cultures of honor' tend to be highly stigmatizing of mental health issues. Cultures of honor place a premium on reputation as an essential feature of personal and collective identity. Honor cultures exist around the world, including Japan as well as the South and Western United States. One far ranging study found striking associations between the honor cultures of these regions of the United States and mental health stigma (Brown et al. 2014). Compared to the North and Eastern United States, the South and Western based honor cultures of the US were more likely to have residents who were concerned that seeking out mental health care suggested personal weakness and affected one's reputation (social stigma) and who, although recognizing mental illness in their family members, were less likely to take them for mental health care (self-stigma). These regions were also less likely to invest public funding in mental health resources and had less mental health practitioners per capita (institutional stigma).

Interventions

It is not unreasonable to suggest, as some have, that mental health professionals have traditionally been lax in taking up the cause of addressing stigma at any level and ought to embrace 'practical stigma management' (Byrne 2000). And, in the abundant literature characterizing the nature of mental health stigma there are emerging ideas about how to address stigma. Chapter 4's framework of the three A's of socioeconomic involvement helps to capture these ideas, as they are readily categorized as either advocacy or activism.

Recall that the global mental health professional who works as an advocate seeks to help change the relevant socioeconomic conditions of individual patients for the better. In the field of stigma reduction, this is embodied in psychoeducational and psycho-therapeutic approaches to self-stigma (Mittal et al. 2012). Psychoeducation seeks to change self-stigmatizing attitudes and has taken the form of print or Internet based information about mental illness in general or specific mental illnesses. It can also involve specialist or peer led group meetings. Psychotherapeutic approaches involve helping patients to cope better with self-stigma via improvements in empowerment, self-esteem, and help seeking and often rely on adaptations of cognitive-behavioral psychotherapy.

Another approach to stigma reduction at the level of individual advocacy involves self-disclosure. Modeled after the successes of the gay rights movement, a 'Coming Out Proud' program has been developed for self-stigmatizing people with mental illness (Corrigan, Kosyluk, & Rusch 2013). This model involves negotiating a menu of gradually more dramatic efforts at self-disclosure and the relative costs and benefits of each (Table 13.1). Global mental health professionals, especially but not necessarily only clinicians, can assist mentally ill patients with weighing the costs and benefits to them of trying any one approach. For example, avoiding social situations (the lowest

Table 13.1 Hierarchy of self-disclosure of mental illness

Social avoidance	Tell no one; avoid situations where illness might be revealed.
Secrecy	Keep illness a secret, but frequent environments with persons with and without mental illnesses.
Selective disclosure	Disclose illness to selected individuals (e.g., coworkers, neighbors).
Indiscriminant disclosure	Do not actively conceal illness from anyone.
Broadcast experience	Actively seek to educate others through sharing personal experience of illness.

Source: Adapted from Corrigan et al. 2013

level in the menu) certainly can shield someone from the effects of public stigma while mitigating the self-consciousness of self-stigma, but it comes at the high price of an insular social life.

On the other hand, the World Health Organization's *Stigma: A Guidebook for Action* promulgates an activist approach to stigma—working at the population level to effect change (WHO 2008). The WHO promotes the idea of a campaign or activity to reduce public stigma and spells out five questions for the global mental health activist to ask in planning this, as follows:

1   Decide about tactics—for example, will the effort involve a media campaign, a project, or lobbying for legal remedies?
2   Choose a level—for example, international, national, local, or even family?
3   Choose a target population(s)—for example, the general population, health professionals, lawmakers, or educators?
4   Decide what mental health problem(s) are the focus—all psychiatric problems or a particular diagnosis?
5   What is the organizing principle(s)—disability rights, human rights/social justice, recovery model, or a biomedical model?

Consumer groups can also serve as a powerful bulwark against stigma (Rusch, Angermeyer, & Corrigan 2005). However, we have found that most countries lack such groups. Activist-oriented global mental health professionals should always explore whether consumer groups exist in a given locality and partner with them where possible. And, if they do not exist, it is worth working with local community members to help establish one.

Conclusions

Mental health stigma proves to be a multi-dimensional problem requiring multiple layers of potential solutions. In our experience, mental health professionals habitually bemoan the unseen forces of stigma arrayed against them and their patients but less habitually characterize the nature of the stigma that they have in mind or formulate a meaningful response. 'Stigma' becomes an ill-defined bogeyman and an unseen enemy, handicapping the possibility for tangible advocacy or activism. In the process, professional hands are wrung over why families, communities, and society do not appreciate the value of mental health care. It is a posture bordering on condescension that we believe can only perpetuate misunderstanding and ignorance about mental illness and mental health.

If global mental health professionals are to reach their goal of improving access to mental health care and maintenance for everyone, everywhere they must render knowledge about mental illness accessible to everyone, everywhere. Psychiatry encompasses a vast field of knowledge about three of the most complex things known to man—the brain, the mind, and the connection between the two. It is also a field about both research ambition and clinical humility and where the questions still far outnumber the answers.

We do not want to unwittingly stigmatize mental health 'non-believers' (some may even be our patients). Therefore we implore all global mental health professionals to incorporate stigma management of some form into their practice, whether at the individual or population level. Unidentified, unaddressed stigma surely begets avoidable suffering, grim psychiatric hospitals, and scarce to non-existent mental health budgets.

To address the 'widespread misunderstanding' about mental illness memorialized by our Belizean nursing students, we recommend you:

✓ Consider anti-stigma work a largely inevitable and integral part of working in any setting where there is not universal access to mental health resources.
✓ Avoid asking *if* there is stigma. Only in a future shaped by a worldwide global mental health campaign can we meaningfully ask the former question and ever expect the answer to be other than affirmative. Instead ask where the stigma is and what form it takes.
✓ Try to be as specific as possible about what you mean by stigma, connecting it with local social and cultural context, specific individuals or populations, and an identifiable impact.
✓ Do not demonize stigma but rather try to understand and even empathize with it. In other words, do not 'stigmatize' people who stigmatize.

References

Alonso, J., Buron, A., Bruffaerts, R., He, Y., Posada-Villa, J., Lepine, J.P., et al. 2008, 'Association of perceived stigma and mood and anxiety disorders: results from the World Mental Health Surveys,' *Acta Psychiatrica Scandinavica*, vol. 118, no. 4, pp. 305–314.

Ando, S., Yamaguchi, S., Aoki, Y., & Thornicroft, G. 2013, 'Review of mental-health-related stigma in Japan,' *Psychiatry and Clinical Neurosciences*, vol. 67, no. 7, pp. 471–482.

Boyd, J.E., Adler, E.P., Otilingam, P.G., & Peters, T. 2014, 'Internalized Stigma of Mental Illness (ISMI) scale: a multinational review,' *Comprehensive Psychiatry*, vol. 55, no. 1, pp. 221–231.

Brown, R.P., Imura, M., & Mayeux, L. 2014, 'Honor and the stigma of mental healthcare,' *Personality and Social Psychology Bulletin*, vol. 40, no. 9, pp. 1119–1131.

Byrne, P. 2000, 'Stigma of mental illness and ways of diminishing it,' *Advances in Psychiatric Treatment*, vol. 6, no. 1, pp. 65–72.

Corrigan, P.W., Kosyluk, K.A., & Rusch, N. 2013, 'Reducing self-stigma by coming out proud,' *American Journal of Public Health*, vol. 103, no. 5, pp. 794–800.

Corrigan, P.W., Watson, A.C., & Barr, L. 2006, 'The self–stigma of mental illness: implications for self–esteem and self–efficacy,' *Journal of Social and Clinical Psychology*, vol. 25, no. 8, pp. 875–884.

Drapalski, A.L., Lucksted, A., Perrin, P.B., Aakre, J.M., Brown, C.H., DeForge, B.R., & Boyd, J.E. 2013, 'A model of internalized stigma and its effects on people with mental illness,' *Psychiatric Services*, vol. 64, no. 3, pp. 264–269.

Ehrlich-Ben Or, S., Hasson-Ohayon, I., Feingold, D., Vahab, K., Amiaz, R., Weiser, M., & Lysaker, P.H. 2013, 'Meaning in life, insight and self-stigma among people with severe mental illness,' *Comprehensive Psychiatry*, vol. 54, no. 2, pp. 195–200.

Gerlinger, G., Hauser, M., De Hert, M., Lacluyse, K., Wampers, M., & Correll, C.U. 2013, 'Personal stigma in schizophrenia spectrum disorders: a systematic review of prevalence rates, correlates, impact and interventions,' *World Psychiatry*, vol. 12, no. 2, pp. 155–164.

Goffman, E. 1963, *Stigma: Notes on the Management of Spoiled Identity*, Simon and Schuster, New York.

Krajewski, C., Burazeri, G., & Brand, H. 2013, 'Self-stigma, perceived discrimination and empowerment among people with a mental illness in six countries: Pan European stigma study,' *Psychiatry Research*, vol. 210, no. 3, pp. 1136–1146.

Livingston, J.D. & Boyd, J.E. 2010, 'Correlates and consequences of internalized stigma for people living with mental illness: a systematic review and meta-analysis,' *Social Science & Medicine*, vol. 71, no. 12, pp. 2150–2161.

Lyons, Z., Laugharne, J., Laugharne, R., & Appiah-Poku, J. 2014, 'Stigma towards mental illness among medical students in Australia and Ghana,' *Academic Psychiatry* (Epub ahead of print).

Mittal, D., Sullivan, G., Chekuri, L., Allee, E., & Corrigan, P.W. 2012, 'Empirical studies of self-stigma reduction strategies: a critical review of the literature,' *Psychiatric Services*, vol. 63, no. 10, pp. 974–981.

Pescosolido, B.A., Medina, T.R., Martin, J.K., & Long, J.S. 2013, 'The "backbone" of stigma: identifying the global core of public prejudice associated with mental illness,' *American Journal of Public Health*, vol. 103, no. 5, pp. 853–860.

Pietrzak, R.H., Johnson, D.C., Goldstein, M.B., Malley, J.C., & Southwick, S.M. 2009, 'Perceived stigma and barriers to mental health care utilization among OEF-OIF veterans,' *Psychiatric Services*, vol. 60, no. 8, pp. 1118–1122.

Rusch, N., Angermeyer, M.C., & Corrigan, P.W. 2005, 'Mental illness stigma: concepts, consequences, and initiatives to reduce stigma,' *European Psychiatry: The Journal of the Association of European Psychiatrists*, vol. 20, no. 8, pp. 529–539.

Vogt, D. 2011, 'Mental health-related beliefs as a barrier to service use for military personnel and veterans: a review,' *Psychiatric Services*, vol. 62, no. 2, pp. 135–142.

World Health Organization 2008. *Stigma: A Guidebook for Action*, Health Scotland, Edinburgh and Glasgow. Available: http://ec.europa.eu/health/mental_health/eu_compass/policy_recommendations_declarations/stigma_guidebook.pdf (accessed December 16, 2014).

Chapter 14

The practice of global mental health

Now imagine yourself in the photo of Sam and his countrymen that has been serving as the departure point for our consideration of global mental health. Think about where you fit in or, for that matter, where you do not. Consider whom you would want to meet; where you would want to work; whom can you help; and whom can you learn from. Maybe you see yourself off frame, in another photo or snapping another photo—helping us to see more of the unseen.

Here we begin to change the perspective. Throughout the book, the dynamic has been one of student and expert, reader and teacher, outsider and insider. In this chapter and the final one that follows, we ask the reader to step into the role of the global mental health professional, hoping the reader who has gotten this far feels that much more equipped and that much more able to see himself or herself doing this work. We mark it as an ending and a beginning.

To synthesize the material in this book and to mobilize the reader to step into the world with Sam, Molly, and the others, we propose a systematic framework for global mental health practice known as the Wheel of Global Mental Health.

The Wheel of Global Mental Health

'The Wheel' consists of seven different elements (Figure 14.1). These are the individual elements that in our experience are the ingredients necessary for launching and running a global mental health program—a program devoted to increasing access to mental health care. As we will soon explain on an item-by-item basis, each element embodies any number of the facts and principles covered in this book. They are arranged as a wheel because of the very practical fact that a change in any one element can affect any of the other elements. Changes—mostly big and even small—can beget a cascade of changes throughout that potentially change the entire face of a global mental health effort. Global mental health work is remarkably and often frustratingly dynamic.

The wheel's seven elements are divided into two categories—those of the *host* and those of the *collaborator*. By 'host' we mean the community in which the global health effort operates. By 'collaborator' we mean the individual from outside that community who seeks to help it address its mental health needs. Global mental health professionals can and must be collaborators and hosts, with the difference hinging on

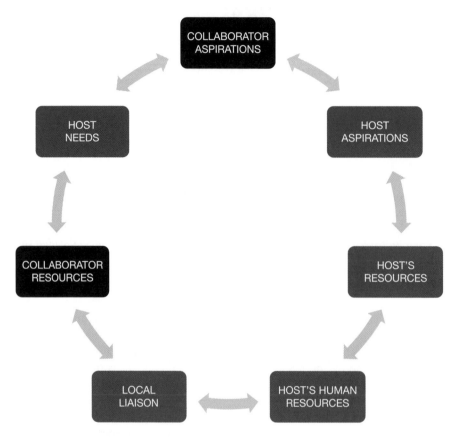

Figure 14.1 The Wheel of Global Mental Health

(grey=host; black=collaborator)

where they live in relation to the community of concern. Nonetheless, we believe that in most low resource settings, whether in the developed or developing word, an 'outsider,' or collaborator, is required to help bring about change in the way mental health issues are brought about.

We have specifically selected the designations of collaborator and host from among any number of ways to frame this relationship (Table 14.1). We wish to avoid a power dynamic that renders one party the 'donor' and the other the 'recipient.' This increasingly outdated way of looking at global relief and development work strikes the wrong tone and makes an erroneous assumption that one party gives and the other receives. One side, the collaborator, necessarily gives more since the other needs more, but it is not mere sentimentality that leads us to say that each side gives and receives in their own ways. If nothing else, the community in need gives to the collaborator(s) an opportunity to be able to help and make a difference. It is for much the same reason that we avoid the axis of 'student' and 'expert.' At the very least, the community side of the equation is expert in its own culture and ways and about the feasibility of proposed solutions. But, it usually goes beyond that, as working in a low

Table 14.1 Defining roles in global mental health

'You'	'Them'
Collaborator	Collaborator
Donor	Recipient
Guest	**Host**
Expert	Student
Westerner	Non-Westerner

resource setting renders many mental health practitioners and planners creative and wily in their approach to problems in ways that those from resource richer settings are not. And, 'Westerner' vs. 'Non-Westerner' simply is a false dichotomy as plenty of Western settings are de facto developing settings when it comes to mental health.

Ultimately, we call the outsider more than a 'guest' since they are not merely visiting but visiting with a professional purpose. They thus become a 'collaborator.' On the other hand, we think the community side is indeed *more* than a collaborator since they are typically thrust into the role of arranging for the accommodations or other logistical and personal needs of the collaborator. We therefore have settled on calling them 'hosts' out of abundant respect for the enormous responsibility they assume for both their community and their collaborators in undertaking a global mental health collaboration.

Therefore, the seven elements of the wheel come out as follows: host needs, host aspirations, host human resources, host non-human resources, collaborator aspirations, collaborator resources, and host liaison. We will explain these item by item.

Host needs

Naturally enough, collaboration around increasing a community's access to mental health care begins with an accounting of its need for mental health care. Ideally, this derives from epidemiological study, data from which may be in the possession of a Ministry of Health, the World Health Organization, or in the scientific literature. However, in many, if not most, low resource settings comprehensive epidemiological data may not be available. And, many such settings may be reluctant to embark on collecting it. Research entails a potential diversion in funding and a delay in service delivery that many overwhelmed localities will not truck.

In practice, then, there are probably two less rigorous but helpful ways to gauge local need. First, it is not unreasonable to extrapolate from existing epidemiological data from nearby or comparable localities or countries (see Chapter 1). Second, your host can tell you what they think is the need. This should involve speaking with multiple 'key informants' about their perception of the need, spanning local mental health professionals or health professionals to schoolteachers to community leaders to 'the man on the street' such as the owner of the hotel where you may be staying. There are certainly rigorous ways of doing this (Biernack & Waldorf 1981) but, again, there may be scant resources or will for doing so, necessitating a more intuitive sampling of local opinions.

Host aspirations

What does your host want? In the practical world of global health, this question could take precedent over what they need. For example, in an overwhelmed low income country, a sole in-country psychiatrist will readily acknowledge and lament how limited or non-existent the public mental health system is across their country. But, they face an immediate problem of overseeing the care of the inpatients at their country's lone and overcrowded psychiatric hospital and might understandably be seeking help with what to do to improve the quality of care and living standards at the hospital.

As mentioned earlier in the book, in our experience the most successful global mental health programs originate with a request from someone or some agency in the host community to the collaborator. Like a patient in clinical practice, they have a 'chief complaint' that may reflect that actual need on the ground, their own views, or both. Their aspirations are a defining element of your collaboration.

However, 'host aspirations' can and should be taken in a broader context. First, a country or community's collective aspirations around mental health may be most concretely embodied in their mental health laws and policies. Assuming such documents exist in some form, they are important to review and become familiar with, possibly in conjunction with meeting relevant government officials. Second, what do identified mental health patients seek for themselves? Answering this may include seeking out information from local patient or 'consumer' advocacy groups if a community is lucky enough to have one. Third, what does the average community member, including health professionals, think about mental health, if at all? This represents an arena where stigma inevitably arises and there are many ways to explore it—via local newspapers, places of worship, schools, businesses, and, again, even at your local accommodations.

Host human resources

Chapter 2 discussed the limited human resources for mental health care delivery worldwide while discussing the different strategies for overcoming this resource 'gap.' In practice, a host's needs and desires must be offset by what they have at their disposal to address them. Gauging local human resources is not usually very complicated and starts with asking about how many mental health professionals are available—psychiatrists, psychologists, social workers, and psychiatric nurses or nurse practitioners. It then extends to potential allies in the health care delivery system—primary care providers and other health care professionals, including not just physicians but also nurses and community health workers. Finally this process can extend to potential new sources for mental health care advocacy and even basic mental health care delivery, such as teachers, spiritual leaders, parents, and other motivated (even unemployed) community members.

Host non-human resources

What tools are available for these human resources to work with? In this part of the Wheel we examine the range of supplies and other items needed for sound mental health practice that were explored in Chapter 3. A careful review of the Wheel could here suggest that an excellent way to help a locality would be to advocate for the government's better stocking the local psychiatric hospital with psychotropic medications listed in WHO's List of Essential Medications. The work, and work satisfaction, of the lone psychiatrist staffing the psychiatric hospital might be most efficiently enhanced by helping them to lobby their government for a steadier supply of basic anti-psychotic medications like haloperidol. A collaborating mental health clinician could step into their clinical role at the hospital to free up the psychiatrist's time to conduct such advocacy, whereas a collaborating public health professional could instead help the situation by doing the advocacy for them.

Collaborator aspirations

What the global mental health collaborator wants to accomplish should be clarified for themselves and their hosts at the outset and re-evaluated throughout as the Wheel spins. There are at least five broad domains in which they may focus their work, as follows: direct care, training/education, advocacy, systems building, and emergency relief. It is recommended that one of these be prioritized according to the ability and interests of the collaborator(s).

The collaborator must also establish the scope of their ambitions. How big of an impact do they need or want to have? Many global mental health professionals would take pride in helping to improve the quality of care at the psychiatric hospital in a low income country whereas some would feel driven to work at the policy level in that country to more systematically address the problems encountered at the hospital and beyond by psychiatric patients.

The ambitions of collaborators need to also be informed by certain facts, and their posture adjusted accordingly. First, however much they and their hosts might seek to replicate the best of Western style mental health care in low resource settings, over 86 percent of research on mental health interventions has been done in high income settings (Patel et al. 2007). And, not only is it possible that these interventions are clinically inappropriate for a given population, but also it is unlikely that they are comparably cost-effective or financially feasible.

Second, there is a school of thought that declares mental health professionals who seek to work in low resource settings to be 'medical imperialists' either naively or malevolently trying to impose Western psychological theories on cultures for which they are neither relevant nor helpful (Summerfield 2008). However strident this position, it may not be far off from the thinking of many people around the world. And, it is worth considering at each turn whether this perspective could sometimes be right.

This raises a final point about the motivations of collaborators in global mental health. Mental health clinicians in particular tend to assess their patients in terms of their 'psychological mindedness,' meaning how open they are to thinking about their problems and needs as having a psychological origin and psychological solution. This makes abundant sense at the individual level for collaborating clinical interventions. But, we should be careful about looking down upon people, or cultures, we see as lacking psychological mindedness. In global mental health work, it may not always be about bringing others up to 'our' level of psychiatric sophistication but rather about figuring out what we can do to better meet different communities and cultures where they are at psychologically.

Collaborator resources

Whatever the global mental health professional may want to do and no matter how welcomed their ambitions may be by their hosts, their own resources will necessarily circumscribe what they can do. They may well want to help transform a given country's outdated mental health policies, but do they have the time or skill set to do this? Given the longitudinal nature of mental health care and its emphasis on care rather than cure, the interests of global mental health practitioners must be sustainable in ways that exceed those of most other global health professionals.

Global mental health practitioners need to be honest with not only themselves but with at least several others about what they can do. First, they should be careful about raising overly optimistic expectations in their hosts. This not only risks being unethical but also can lead to burnout.

Second, at this point in time we know of very few people who are full time global mental health professionals outside of colleagues working in research. In fact, there may be reason to argue that global mental health professionals should always retain a base of clinical or other activities in their home communities if for no other reason than to stay current with innovations as well as connected to streams of personnel and funding that can bolster their efforts. Either way, the current reality means that global mental health professionals must take themselves away from patients, other day-to-day work commitments, and/or family and friends. Patients, colleagues, employers, family, and friends should have a say in how much time and resources a global mental health professional can commit to other communities. In a very real way, they are contributing, too.

Host liaison

Finally, the seventh element of the Wheel is the 'liaison,' the individual(s) in the host community who is the primary contact and partner for the collaborator. In fact, it would not be a stretch to say that they really belong at the hub of the Wheel. Typically, this would be the very person who saw an unmet mental health need and undertook to do something about it, in the process requesting help from the collaborator. Over and over again we have found that this person is so vital to the success of a global mental health program that it can (and does) collapse without them. As they live in the low resource setting and the collaborator usually can only be there part-time, they have primary responsibility for promoting and sustaining it on a regular basis.

We do not know of any way to readily identify and recruit such a person. As we said, they usually 'self-identify.' But, in inauspicious cases where they must be sought, here are their usual characteristics—charismatic, tireless, reliable, humble, and Internet-savvy.

Conclusions

The Wheel of Global Mental Health provides a broad strategy for practicing global mental health rather than a step-by-step formula for doing so. A more tactical approach to its implementation is presented for the reader's consideration in the Appendix.

For now, we leave the reader with a few last suggestions as they pivot towards global mental health practice:

✓ If you are setting up a new global mental health program, try to fill in what you have and what you need for addressing all seven items of the Wheel. Again, refer to the Appendix for help with doing this.
✓ If you are joining an ongoing global mental health program, try to understand it from the perspective of the Wheel. This will give you a comprehensive view of the work you are about to embark on.
✓ Whether working in a new or ongoing mental health program, try to identify the most fragile parts of the Wheel and see if you can focus your efforts there.
✓ As all parts of the Wheel bear on one another, anticipate that any global mental health program is a dynamic and ever changing entity. Changes in goals, personnel, funding, or other resources inevitably have ramifications, sometimes for the better and sometimes not.

References

Biernack, P. & Waldorf, D. 1981, 'Snowball sampling: problems and techniques of chain referral sampling,' *Sociological Methods & Research*, vol. 10, no. 2, pp. 141–163.
Patel, V., Araya, R., Chatterjee, S., Chisholm, D., Cohen, A., De Silva, M., et al. 2007, 'Treatment and prevention of mental disorders in low-income and middle-income countries,' *The Lancet*, vol. 370, no. 9591, pp. 991–1005.
Summerfield, D. 2008, 'How scientifically valid is the knowledge base of global mental health?' *British Medical Journal (Clinical research edn.)*, vol. 336, no. 7651, pp. 992–994.

Chapter 15

The experience of global mental health

Why isn't there a mental health professional in the newspaper image? There are many reasons for this hinted at elsewhere in this book, including their sheer scarcity and the widespread stigma in most places around mental illness. Both factors conspire to limit the presence, the visibility, and even the marketability of mental health professionals. It can be especially daunting for the global mental health professional to step into this vacuum. On the other hand, it is precisely this vacuum that necessitates their doing just that—stepping into the picture.

In Chapter 13, we reviewed *how* to step into Sam's world as a global mental health professional. Here we conclude the book by discussing *what* it is like to step into the picture. To do so, we draw from our own experience working in the United States, Central America and the Caribbean, sub-Saharan Africa, and Asia. We highlight this diversity because we hope and believe it lends generalizability to our observations and compensates for the absence of any research underpinning to what we advise. Some of what follows should even be generalizable to global health practice as whole. Either way, we hope it sufficiently conveys to the emerging global mental health professional what being on the ground in a low resource setting is like and therefore helps them assess their personal and professional readiness for the work.

Arrival

What are you doing when you arrive? Mostly we fly to destinations like Sam's country. So, after your airplane lands and you disembark, collect your luggage, and pass through customs, the prescribed and the familiar come to an end. Propelled by your aspirations and an airplane, you have been thrust out into the host country beyond the doors of the airport and are finally born a global mental health professional. You must now navigate in a new world.

The most important thing to know before any trip is how you will get to your local accommodations. This of course involves having arranged for your accommodations in advance, something that your hosts or the organization you are working with may have done for you. As for getting there, this too may have been arranged. Many partnering agencies are happy to pick up and drive you after such a long journey. If so, be sure to get the name and contact information for the driver. But, if not, be sure you chart out in advance how you plan to travel locally.

The first day

Where are you going to report on the first day of your work? We all have our work routines, and where we are going to show up on the first day of the work week is not in doubt, whether it is our office, hospital, school, or organization. Knowing where to go on the first day therefore often slips the minds of global mental health professionals until they are ready for bed on the eve of beginning to work.

Before you leave home we recommend picturing in your mind where you will be on your first morning of work and how you will get there. In part this is a logistical question since you are out of your routine. It is also an emotional one, as reflection prepares you as well as anything for anticipating the experience to follow. But, it is also an organizational question that provides an invaluable check on the adequacy of your work plan. If the question surprises you, then either your plan is vague or your familiarity with it is lacking. If in reviewing your plan you are still unclear, the time to hone it is well before you leave. Not knowing what you will be doing on your first day may be a very clear signal that the vision for your trip needs to be re-visited.

What you will be doing on your first day should usually boil down to whom you will be meeting with. If you refer to the prior chapter on the Wheel of Global Mental Health, this is usually the local liaison—the person, usually a local mental health professional, with which you have been working to organize and plan the trip in the first place. The first day is usually an orientation to them, the mental health system, and ideally the community. Many professionals expect to 'work' on their first day, but in this case working means meeting, greeting, and learning.

We recommend that you pack your knapsack or day travel bag with several key items. First, be sure you have some bottled water, hand sanitizer, toilet tissue, and snacks such as granola bars. In the hustle and bustle of the first day and especially in places where stores and restaurants as you usually know them are in short supply, you may not have ready access to lunch and may not want to obligate your hosts to have to think about this for you. Second, bring a notebook and pen or an electronic device on which you can take lots of notes. No matter how much you prepared before traveling, you will be greeted with a barrage of new information and new faces. Third, bring business cards that include your email address. In some places, it is custom to introduce yourself with your business card, whereas in others it is simply a way for people to see you as professional and eager to stay in touch. Fourth, have a camera or smartphone with at least still photography capability (see later section on photography). Finally, you should have a gift(s) on hand for your hosts. Before you leave home, think about bringing them something from your home institution or your city or community. You might even ask them whether there is something you can bring them or their organization. For example, once some colleagues asked us to bring DVDs of popular movies that touched on mental health issues for use as psycho-educational tools.

The second day

What happens next? A major part of your first day of working in-country should involve discussing the plan for your trip with your hosts. Sometimes you may be provided with a day-by-day schedule without asking. In all likelihood, you will want one. Mental health clinicians in particular are accustomed to tightly scheduled days based on patient hours and other commitments. However, depending upon the nature of your work in the host community, this may not be feasible.

Consider the following projects and how differently they lend themselves to rigorous scheduling:

1   A group of public health and medical students arrive in Sam's country with the goal of setting up alcohol self-help groups modeled on AA (see Chen et al. 2014 for details of one such effort). Supported by the Ministry of Health, they plan to recruit key stakeholders in several pilot communities, conduct focus groups, and then begin to roll out self-help groups based on the input of these focus groups. At the end of their two months in-country, they hope to have one such group functioning and showing signs of sustainability.

2   A psychiatrist arrives in Sam's country with the goal of supervising public health nurses as they integrate mental health into their practice in the district health clinics scattered throughout the country. In this pilot phase and with only one supervising psychiatrist, it was decided to focus on five clinics in adjacent districts outside of the capital.

Scenario 1 does not lend itself to daily scheduling from the outset. There are too many variables to be able to say exactly when and where the focus groups can be held as the students first need to recruit focus group members, hold the groups, analyze the information, and deploy what they learn to initiate the self-help groups. At best, their hosts may be able to pre-arrange meetings with, for example, the senior public health nurse in each community as a starting point for recruiting focus group members. Otherwise, a scenario like this lends itself to a weekly timeline which the global mental health professional establishes and then modifies with the input of their hosts on their first day or so in-country. And, we have found that over time a daily schedule does emerge as a project like this gains momentum, sometimes to an overwhelming degree.

On the other hand, Scenario 2 should lend itself nicely to daily scheduling from the outset. If there are five clinics and the psychiatrist plans to be in-country for four weeks, then rotating to one per day each week will enable them to work with each clinic's nursing staff four times across their stay. If that is deemed too little or traveling to a different clinic every day of the week is impractical due to the distances involved and availability of transport, then one clinic can be dropped and they can spend a full week at each of the four clinics. In this scenario, the global mental health professional should expect a schedule to be drawn up in advance by their hosts.

Regardless of the feasibility of working out a schedule, a critical point is that many host countries and cultures operate with less emphasis on precise scheduling than do the countries from which most global mental health professionals hail. Meetings may begin late or be canceled outright for reasons that may baffle an outsider. We are in no position to parse the cross-cultural anthropology of time management. But, we can say that a flexible nature is essential in global health work of any kind.

In-country schedule changes constitute a reality that global mental health professionals may chafe at. Two things can be said about this. First, it is certainly the case that some health, mental health, and public health professionals are therefore not well suited to global health work. This is not a moral failing and is actually advantageous—after all, someone must 'hold down the fort' back home while others scatter abroad.

Second, the uncertainties around time inherent in much of global mental health work hold a clue as to the nature of that work. Clinicians in particular who seek to provide clinical care are likely to experience the most frustration over schedule changes since they have limited, if any, time for follow-up of patients whom they have newly met. On the other hand, clinicians who see themselves as teachers of in-country providers will have more flexibility since mental health teaching, training, and supervision inherently have a more sustained impact. In example two above, consider how providing a single hour of individual teaching and modeling with one public health nurse about how to assess suicidality in one of their patients should have more of an impact than assessing the suicidality directly. Substantial involvement in direct clinical care generally only makes sense when the collaborating mental health clinician plans to stay for months if not a year or more (one exception is providing clinical care when the usual local provider is temporarily unable to due to vacation or other personal reasons).

Journaling

For both personal and professional reasons, we strongly recommend that global mental health professionals keep a daily journal that they would feel comfortable having colleagues and future missioners read. This can be a written or electronic journal or even a blog. Seeing new places, meeting new people, and learning new ways of doing things ensures that you will face a barrage of new experiences and information well beyond day one. And, you will have to process and retain all of this while acclimating to be away from home and potentially in a foreign culture.

Journals afford the global mental health professional an opportunity to reflect and a much better chance of remembering. The narrative style of journaling means they can also be an evocative means of orienting future travellers. With proper re-formatting, their content could also be turned into reports for one's agency or funding source.

The personal nature of journaling argues against dictating their format, and yet a relatively uniform format will help ensure their utility for others. We also find that many people want some guidance on what to include. We therefore suggest referring back to the Wheel of Global Mental Health (see Chapter 13) and using the seven parts of the Wheel to organize one's thoughts. Each journal entry can then be divided into two main parts and associated elements: Host—Needs, Human and Other Resources, Aspirations and Liaison; and Collaborator—Aspirations and Resources. It need not be the case that all seven elements receive attention on a given day, but the global mental health journalist should at least reflect on each at the end of every work day in the field and document accordingly. Ask, 'What did I learn today about {fill in with an item from the Wheel}?' Each entry should then conclude with a 'Follow-Up' section that documents action items in support of current programming or ideas for future programming. See Box 15.1 for a sample journal entry.

**BOX 15.1.   A SAMPLE JOURNAL ENTRY FOR
A PSYCHIATRIST SUPERVISING PUBLIC HEALTH
NURSES IN SAM'S COUNTRY**

Date: May 12, 2012

Host

Needs—*In clinic today, I was struck by how many cases of somatization the nurse sees. It was clear to me from reviewing their charts that their physical complaints have actually been worked up well and found lacking an organic etiology. The nurse seems completely at a loss as to what to do with them.*

Non-Human Resources—*It turns out the nurses can get blood alcohol levels if their patient is willing to go to a private lab and pay out of pocket.*

Liaison—*Met a wonderful priest who has been trying to teach himself motivational interviewing to help his alcohol abusing parishioners.*

Collaborator

Aspirations—*I am beginning to wonder how much I can really accomplish this month and wonder if I need to reassess the plan, if not our entire strategy here. There is too much to do!*

Follow-up

1   *Review the literature on somatization across cultures.*
2   *Be sure to email Father Hull when back in the US so that we can provide him with more help with motivational literature. Get him a book or access to an online course?*
3   *Email the program director back in the US to review the feasibility of our plan.*

Photography

Photos complement journals. Usual mental health practice or research in well-resourced settings generally does not lend itself to casual photography. The face-to-face interactions of clinical work or the minutiae of research are not especially dramatic or photogenic. And, both clinical and clinical research encounters are of course shrouded in confidentiality. However, global mental work can be uniquely dramatic and should be captured on film so long as it is done respectfully and ethically.

The journal of the global mental health professional should reflect their passion for ensuring better allocation of resources for mental health care worldwide. But, 'a picture is worth a thousand words.' Photos of dilapidated psychiatric hospitals, of the earnest professionals who staff them, or of patients who inhabit them can powerfully convey a message that helps to mobilize policymakers, attract funding, and recruit other mental health and public health professionals to join the global mental health movement.

In rare instances, a professional photographer may be able to assist a global mental health team. And, a powerful if labor-intensive research method known as Photovoice allows 'subjects' to document their own lives in photos and narrative (Wang 1999). More often than not, though, it will be left to the global mental health Professional to also serve as photographer and journalist. Whoever the photographer and notwithstanding the eventual quality of the photos, we offer a few guidelines for deferentially capitalizing on photographic opportunities:

1   Always have a camera with you.
2   Always ask before taking any pictures, including inquiring about policies on photography if you are visiting an institution or hospital.
3   Remind hosts how photos can amplify advocacy efforts for mental health needs in-country and back home, but be sure to do so diplomatically and without strong-arming.
4   Try to take photos of objects (i.e. a Ministry of Health's poster about its mental health mission), structures (i.e., an inpatient psychiatric ward), or even parts of people other than their faces where possible.
5   If you want to take a picture of someone, especially a patient, always ask him or her and be sure they are able to provide informed consent.
6   Always carry consent forms if you anticipate using photos of people for future publication of any kind.
7   Do not forget that you have your camera and that it is a tool of your work.

Recreation

Many global health projects operate in far-flung places filled with unique culture and beauty. Colleagues or students sometimes ask us whether it is okay to take time off to sightsee. The answer: not only is it acceptable for all global health professionals to entertain their natural curiosity and need for leisure, it is essential that global mental health professionals do so.

In the biopsychosocial model that underpins modern psychiatric practice, we look at the whole person and see their mental health and their mental illness as a composite of their biology, their psychology, and their social circumstances (Engel 1980). Parachuting into health clinics to supervise nurses around their approach to mental health will fail biopsychosocially if the global mental health professional does not have some personal acquaintance with what life is like for the patients who walk in the clinic door.

For example, it is one thing to advise the nurse about how to counsel patients who misuse alcohol. It is an entirely different thing to walk the streets of the town and see how many little roadside bars there are and how much socializing goes on around them. Even if a patient expresses sincere concern about how their drinking has yielded abnormal liver function results, what help is offered to them for finding a new way of socializing and even a new social circle in a setting where drinking is how so many people spend their leisure time?

Of course, travel to tourist attractions may not afford a significant chance to see what life is like in a new community or country. But, it certainly has its place in helping to paint the cultural, social, and historical context in which 'foreigners' find themselves. Importantly, it helps to ensure that the focus of global mental health efforts is not the mentally ill who are Sam's countrymen and women but rather are Sam's countrymen and women who have mental illness or who deserve to have every chance to maintain their mental health.

Conclusion

For those of us lucky enough to have the chance to participate in global mental health work, capturing the experience can often escape words. One pre-medical student who accompanied us on a recent trip to Central America said of her first experience what we struggle with all of the time: 'This was one of the most amazing experiences of my life. Everyone back home keeps asking me what exactly we are doing here. But, you know, they couldn't possibly understand.' We hope this chapter and this book have helped you to better understand.

References

Chen, A., Smart, Y., Morris-Patterson, A., & Katz, C. 2014, 'Piloting alcohol self-help groups in Saint Vincent/Grenadines,' *Annals of Global Health,* vol. 80, no. 2, pp. 83–88.

Engel, G.L. 1980, 'The clinical application of the biopsychosocial model,' *The American Journal of Psychiatry,* vol. 137, no. 5, pp. 535–544.

Wang, C.C. 1999, 'Photovoice: a participatory action research strategy applied to women's health,' *Journal of Women's Health,* vol. 8, no. 2, pp. 185–192.

Appendix
Scaling up

Karen Carpio Barrantes

Here we present a practical approach to scaling up mental health services in low resource settings. It is based on the Model for Psychosocial Care Delivery (Carpio Barrantes 2014). This Model was recently conceived to assist program planners and decision makers in low-resource settings in the process of scaling up packages of mental health care such as the mhGAP Program and Intervention Guide (mhGAP-IG) (WHO 2008, 2010). It was developed by synthesizing findings from the literature and interviews with global mental health experts from around the globe. The Model is organized according to the seven components of Wheel of Global Mental Health presented in Chapter 14 of this book. In addition, an independent component for contextual considerations has been included.

This algorithm for scaling up represents the tactical counterpart to the strategies embodied in the Wheel of Global Mental Health. If the photo of Sam and his countrymen poses a puzzle about how to provide mental health care in low-resource settings and this book then de-constructs that puzzle, what follows provides an array of pieces with which to solve it. As in the Model for Psychosocial Care Delivery, we present a series of 'Decision Points' with tables that contain menus of options highlighting recommendations and considerations for scaling up.

Contextual considerations

Gathering general contextual information increases chances for success when scaling up mental health services in low-resource settings (Samuel et al. 2015; Eaton et al. 2011, p. 1600). The elements of the proposed contextual analysis do not encompass any decision points (Table A.1).

1 Host's needs

Most localities will be unable to address all nine mental health disorders identified as priorities in the mhGAP-IG. Absent this ideal, epidemiological studies that evaluate morbidity, mortality, and disability due to specific mental health disorders can inform program planners and allow them to make decisions about budget allocation that maximize the impact of mental health services. However, these studies are very time-consuming and very costly in financial and technical terms. In reality, most low-resource settings lack such data and end up making decisions

Table A.1 Contextual analysis

General contextual considerations usually present in low resource settings
– Mental health is not seen as a public health priority in most low resource settings.
– Budget allocation for mental health care services is usually insufficient.
– Most mental health care services are offered in outdated long-stay, specialized care facilities.
– Integrating mental health care into general health care has proved to be very challenging.
– Adequately trained human resources for mental health care are scarce.
– Care providers are not always up to date with current evidence-based treatments and tools for mental health care provision.

Contextual analysis essentials
– Health system and mental health system organization.
– Social, economic, and political context.
– Local culture and values related to mental health and mental health care.
– Educational level of the population.
– Stigma related to mental and substance use disorders (in the population and among health professionals).

that affect budget allocation without really knowing which conditions are most burdensome.

➲ *Decision Point: Identifying the target population*

Program planners and local stakeholders have to decide which is going to be their target population, and whether they will prioritize investment for a specific disorder or set of disorders (i.e. as recommended by the mhGAP-IG), for a specific population (i.e. more vulnerable populations), or if mental health services will be provided without diagnostic distinction. These variables amount to four different options (Table A.2).

Minimally, we recommend focusing efforts on improving access to care for people with depressive disorders (option D), which is estimated to be the leading cause of disability globally (WHO 2001) and to be accountable for the highest proportion of disease burden attributable to mental and substance use disorders across all regions considered in GBD 2010 (IHME 2013, p. 6; WHO 2001) accounting for 40.5 percent (31.7–49.2) of DALY caused by mental and substance use disorders (Whiteford & Baxter 2013, p. 1582).

Also, ethical aspects of prioritizing care at non-specialized health settings should be addressed by making sure that all the population has access to mental health services at one level or another.

2 Host's aspirations

Two axes constitute the host's aspirations component of the Wheel of Global Mental Health: Axis I concerns improving mental health awareness and Axis II considers

Table A.2 Identifying the target population

Define target population			
A	B	C	D
No prioritizing: Provide mental health care to all people seeking care at non-specialized health settings without diagnostic distinction.	Prioritize a population or populations with a specific mental disorder according to identified local needs: Consider that the mhGAP-IG prioritizes nine psychiatric disorders for treatment at non-specialized health settings: depressive disorders, schizophrenia and other psychotic disorders, suicide, epilepsy, dementia, alcohol use disorders, substance use, and mental disorders in children.	Prioritize vulnerable populations according to: health condition, socio-economic status, geography, gender, age, ethnicity, disability status, risk status related to sex and gender, or other populations identified to be at-risk for health disparities.	Start by prioritizing depressive disorders and add other conditions as resources become available.

how to improve access to care. Both axes are interrelated since local stakeholders and care providers need to be aware of the burden of psychiatric disorders in their locality in order to understand and be willing to improve access to care.

Axis I: improving mental health awareness

Lack of political support poses one of the main barriers to scaling up mental health care in low-resource settings (Eaton et al. 2011, p. 1594). Fostering awareness of the immense personal, societal, and economic burden of mental disorders is key to successfully scaling up mental health services (Carpio Barrantes 2014; Lancet Global Mental Health Group et al. 2007).

➲ *Decision Point 1: Identifying key stakeholders*

A menu of options of possible key stakeholders to whom direct global mental health activism around scaling up follows in Table A.3.

➲ *Decision Point 2: Defining methods to foster awareness*

A menu of key messages and methods that could be used to convince decision makers, funders, and other stakeholders about the need for scaling up mental health services follows in Table A.4.

Table A.3 Identifying key stakeholders

Key stakeholders and decision makers for mental health care improvement

- Regional and local government decision makers (i.e. Ministry of Health, Public Health administration, municipalities).
- Mental health specialists providing care at private or public specialized settings.
- General care providers working at non-specialized health settings.
- Community associations, grassroots organizations, worker unions, health or social foundations linked to the health sector.
- Service users and their families.

Table A.4 Fostering mental health awareness

Key messages to foster mental health awareness

- There is no health without mental health.
- Stigma and discrimination lead to pervasive human rights violations against people with psychiatric disorders.
- The global burden of disease of mental disorders is great, and low resource settings are especially vulnerable.
- The cost of time-lost in general care medical practice due to the lack of knowledge of non-specialized health providers about mental health care is high.
- The delivery of evidence-based brief and simple psychosocial interventions by general care providers improves access to care in a cost-effective way.

Methods to foster awareness in low-resource settings

- Use of media: billboards, television, or radio spots.
- Use existing websites as platforms for information and training.
- Plan workshops for different target populations (users and professionals).
- Use existing health professional societies as platforms to reach stakeholders.
- Establish a mental health association for training and awareness efforts.
- Use posters and short films to create community awareness.
- Develop mental health community awareness campaigns or festivals.

Axis II: improving access to mental health care

A series of decisions must be made to ensure access to mental health care in low resource settings. Five Decision Points are proposed to assist program planners in key issues regarding improving access to psychosocial care.

➲ *Decision Point 1: Reorganizing mental health care (Table A.5)*

➲ *Decision Point 2: Defining the health setting*

When intending to improve access to mental health care in non-specialized health settings, planners have to start by defining the health setting for care provision. We recommend selecting the most abundant and geographically widespread type of

Table A.5 Reorganizing mental health care

General recommendations for mental health care reorganization

- Consider that systems have a hard time changing at an individual and systems level.
- Make sure care provision reorganization is initiated by a need or aspiration of the host community.
- Getting buy-in from countries and local settings and having them be in charge of efforts improves chances for program sustainability.
- Having a very motivated and committed person in charge of running the efforts is key.
- Identify other entities and programs providing psychosocial services to the population before creating new ones.
- When possible do not add new programs and staff and do use existing health programs as modifiable platforms to meet mental health needs.
- Find health programs that have proven to be successful locally and replicate them at new settings.
- Look beyond the health sector to coordinate actions with agencies from other sectors (education, social).
- Plan in advance strategies to overcome known barriers and be prepared for unexpected obstacles when scaling up mental health care.
- Pre-set manageable goals with measurable outcomes for each specific health setting.
- Provide on-site technical support to local stakeholders with no experience scaling up health programs.
- Strengthen relationships between primary, secondary, and tertiary levels of care.
- Ensure sufficient human resources at each health facility to cover all aspects of care.
- Rely on support and supervision by mental health experts available at other facilities and levels of care.
- Explore all possible organizational structures for a mental health program to find an option that responds to local needs and resource availability (i.e. individual care or group care).
- Increase outpatient services to decentralize services from specialized health facilities.
- Provide care via house visits in case no physical space is available at the primary care facility.
- Use phone technology to provide care.

non-specialized health setting available at community level that has proven to be sustainable over time (Table A.6).

➲ *Decision point 3: Choosing mental health care services*

Whether intending to scale up an entire package of mental health care such as the mhGAP-IG or just a part of it, non-pharmacological/psychosocial interventions should possess certain characteristics in order to be feasible and affordable in low resource settings (Table A.7).

➲ *Decision Point 4: Screening*

Low cost approaches to screening for psychiatric disorders entails the use of non-proprietary, freely accessible screening tools that are not time consuming and for

Table A.6 Defining the health setting

Possible health settings for mental health care provision	
A Public sector	B Private sector
Primary care clinics Community clinics School based clinics Mobile clinics Home visits Outpatient services Day care centers Telemedicine Outreach clinics	

Table A.7 Choosing mental health care services

Non-pharmacological and psychosocial interventions' suggested characteristics
− Should be brief. − Should be specific. − Should be contextually appropriate. − Should be culturally relevant. − Should be delivered in the local language. − Should address the community's interests. − Should be easy to deliver for general care providers. − Should address stigma related to psychiatric disorders. − Should address both psychological and social components of care. − Should be provided even when medication is not available. − Should ensure the respect of human rights. − Should address the patient's general needs, other than medical treatment. − Should inform users about common questions, problems, and coping strategies for illness related situations.

which highly specialized human resources are not required. Table A.8 gives a list of considerations in deciding if and how to conduct screenings.

➲ *Decision Point 5: Defining clear referral pathways*

Several key strategies for optimizing mental health referral pathways between various care settings follow in Table A.9.

3 Host's human resources

A range of human resources could be used to provide mental health care in low resource settings. We have organized them into three categories as shown in Figure A.1.

Table A.8 Screening

Screening tool considerations

– Should be brief.
– Should be easy to use for available human resources.
– Should be inexpensive to obtain and use on a regular basis.
– Should be contextually appropriate.
– Should be validated for the local health setting.
– Should be sensitive to identify signs and symptoms of target mental disorders.
– Should address violence screening (sexual and physical).
– Should consider different levels of education, including illiteracy.

Table A.9 Defining clear referral pathways

Strategies to optimize referral pathways

– Establish a single entry point to the health care system.
– Establish a case severity scale for targeted mental disorders and use it for referral purposes.
– Establish clear referral pathways between general care providers and mental health specialists.
– General care providers should refer patients to a more specialized level only if the patient needs more specialized care that he or she is not trained to provide.
– Before referring, the general care practitioner should consult with the specialist when doubting about the need for referral (via phone or email), until the general care provider is confident to make the decision on his or her own.
– Define the roles and responsibilities of general care providers and mental health specialists according to case severity.
– Develop channels to build good relationships between care providers at all levels of care.
– The same patient should see the same care provider on a regular basis to ensure treatment continuity and to build a therapeutic alliance.
– Identify other entities and programs providing services that can serve as support to the population with mental disorders and create clear and simple communication pathways for easy referral.

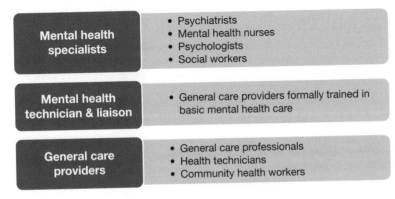

Figure A.1 Mental health workforce

➲ *Decision Point 1: Redefining human resources: roles and responsibilities*

There should be an ongoing mutual relationship among mental health specialists, general care providers, and the mental health technician or liaison (Figure A.2; Table A.10).

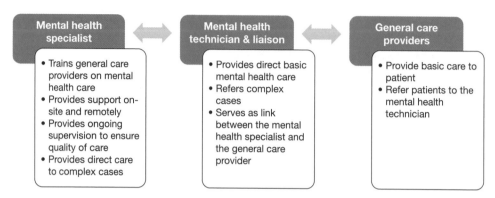

Figure A.2 Redefining human resources: roles and responsibilities

Table A.10 Human resources task menu

Mental health specialists' suggested tasks

− Shift the role of mental health specialists at non-specialized settings from providing care to patients to being responsible for:
   o program development and coordination,
   o training, support, and supervision of general care providers working at non-specialized health settings,
   o assessment and management of complex cases.
− Social workers can be responsible for addressing the concrete needs of patients.

General care providers and health technicians' suggested tasks

− General care professionals can be responsible for diagnosis and pharmacological treatment of psychiatric disorders depending on local regulations.
− General doctors can focus on diagnosis and prescribing psychiatric medication.
− Nursing staff (different specialization levels) are a great resource for patient and family psychoeducation.
− Nursing staff and health technicians can be used to provide basic psychosocial care.

Health technicians and community health workers' suggested tasks

− Identify people with mental disorders signs and symptoms within the community and refer them to the primary care clinic for mental health assessment and management.
− Screen patients at non-specialized health facilities.
− Provide basic mental health care in the community or at non-specialized health facilities.
− Refer patients to other mental health services available.
− Support general care professionals with basic care provision tasks to optimize their time.
− Improve access to care in remote areas.
− Peers can educate people with mental disorders about their illness.

⮕ *Decision Point 2: Defining the strategy to obtain human resources*

Here are potential approaches for establishing sustainable human resources at low resource settings (Tables A.11 and A.12).

Table A.11 Defining a strategy to obtain human resources

Strategies to obtain human resources	
Establish organizational change	Establish a new program
Funds need to be allocated temporarily, until change in the organization is established.	New funding is necessary on a long-term basis to ensure sustainability.

Organizational change is less costly than establishing a new program.
Do not add new staff unless sufficient funding for training, support,
and supervision is available.

A	B
Reorganization of current human resources	**Recruitment of new human resources**
If mental health specialists and general care providers are available within the health system, then their roles and responsibilities need to be redefined to optimize the resource.	If there are no mental health specialists, mental health technicians, or general care providers available, then new human resources need to be recruited.
1 Budgeting mental health specialists' time to provide training and supervision to general care providers and mental health technicians.	1 Recruiting already trained mental health providers (either specialists or technicians).
2 Budgeting time and financial resources for training of general care providers on basic mental health care.	2 Recruiting untrained general care providers (professionals, technicians, or community health workers) and train them to become mental health technicians.

Table A.12 Low-cost sustainable human resources

Recommendations for obtaining sustainable human resources at low cost
– Diversify the workforce.
– Recruit and train general care providers already providing general care at non-specialized health settings.
– Take advantage of human resources already trained in psychosocial care for specific health programs (i.e. HIV-AIDS).
– Identify the roles that peers, family, and community agents can have in providing mental health care.
– Have general care providers work in teams to share the workload.
– Shift the tasks of specialists working at the tertiary and secondary level to provide training and support at the primary level.
– When recruiting new staff for mental health care select people who can commit mid to long term.

Table A.12 Continued

Recommendations for obtaining sustainable human resources at low cost

- Using volunteers to provide mental health care is not a sustainable strategy because of high turnover and 'brain drain.' Some kind of compensation, even if small, needs to be given for the workforce to be sustained (i.e. stipend, academic credit, traveling expenses).
- Reduce specialists' transportation and accommodation costs by using communication technology for remote support and supervision.
- If available select community health workers and general care professionals who:
  o show an inclination to work in the mental health field,
  o are empathetic,
  o have good communication and networking skills,
  o have at least basic academic knowledge (i.e. reading and writing skills),
  o have cultural competence.
- Train high school graduates to become mental health providers.
- Partner with existing NGOs, hospitals, or other collaborators who already employ mental health specialists and who would be willing to contribute their time.
- If new staff are added specifically for mental health care at a health facility, original general care staff should be included in their training so that they understand their roles and value.

⮕ *Decision Point 3: Training, support, and supervision*

Here are specific strategies for training, supporting, and supervising human resources (Table A.13).

Table A.13 Human resources development platform for mental health care

Strategies to build a human resources development platform for mental health care

- Train existing personnel in mental health care provision to reduce the cost of hiring new staff.
- Use existing training, support, and supervision channels available for general health care and use them for mental health care.
- Make sure that the budget covers the three aspects of the human resource development platform (training, support, and supervision) in an ongoing way to ensure sustainability.
- Distribute tasks among trainers: use psychiatrists to provide training in pharmacotherapy and psychologists and social workers to provide training in psychosocial care.
- Provide training for local care providers to become mental health care trainers so that the workforce can continue to expand locally.
- Use training methods that will provide general care providers with a sense of familiarity and confidence about managing patients with mental disorders, such as:
  o combining on-site and remote trainings,
  o doing supervised patient-interviewing with patients,
  o practicing with role plays,
  o using videos to exemplify the population and interventions,
  o using case study methodology.
- Combine on-site and remote training, support, and supervision.
- Provide protocols, guidelines, and other resources that are requested by primary care providers to facilitate their job.

Table A.13 Continued

Strategies to build a human resources development platform for mental health care

- Create mental health providers' group meetings to share experiences and ensure peer support.
- Create a local mental health assembly composed of all mental health care providers that meets regularly for training and awareness activities.
- Ensure easy access to mental health specialists by the general care providers in charge of basic mental health care (i.e. via phone, email, chat, other communication platform).
- Create a structure for support and supervision of mental health programs (i.e. networks or teams of mental health specialists that oversee several mental health programs at primary care clinics).
- Use technology to provide remote access training, support, and supervision in order to reduce transportation and professionals' time (i.e. web based training).

Now here is a list of contents for basic mental health training (Table A.14).

Table A.14 Basic mental health training

Specific contents for basic mental health training

- Prevalence of mental disorders in non-specialized health settings.
- Understanding mental disorders as a psychological, social, and biological disorder.
- Public health capacity for mental health care providers and program coordinators.
- Disability caused by mental disorders.
- How to differentiate between mental illness and physical illness when a patient is agitated.
- Patient assessment and diagnosis with basic screening tools and clinical interviewing.
- Structuring a treatment plan for people with mental disorders.
- Effective use of the mhGAP-IG.
- Responsibilities and limitations as non-specialized mental health care providers.
- Well-timed referral to more specialized services.
- How non-specialized mental health care providers can effectively support general care doctors.
- Delivery of basic psychosocial intervention techniques:
  o shared principles of psychosocial care for treating mental disorders (i.e. mhGAPs general principles for care),
  o active listening techniques,
  o counseling techniques,
  o creating a therapeutic alliance,
  o managing counter transference,
  o psychological first aid,
  o managing frustration with non-compliant patients.
- According to needs and resources more advanced interventions such as Cognitive Behavioral Therapy, Interpersonal Therapy, Psychodynamic Psychotherapy, or interventions for specific vulnerable populations (i.e. child mental health) can be taught to general care providers.

4 Host's non-human resources

In order for human resources to be able to effectively scale up mental health services or evidence based packages of care for psychiatric disorders, adequate *non-human resources* must also be present.

➲ *Decision Point 1: Identifying other resources needed*

Here is a list of non-human resources that are necessary for scaling up mental health care (Table A.15).

➲ *Decision Point 2: Obtaining other resources*

This menu of low cost strategies for obtaining non-human resources (Table A.16) can help to fill in gaps identified in Table A.15.

Table A.15 Identifying other resources needed

Basic non-human resources for mental health care
Infrastructure

– Social services agencies and services.
– Space:
  o private room or space for counseling,
  o conference room for family and staff meetings.
– Administrative infrastructure (i.e. for registration of patients).

Technical
– Library access. – Access to good quality and sensitive screening tools. – Educational pamphlets and posters for mental health education. – Basic books, guidelines, compilations, and materials for basic mental health care and psychosocial care. – Equipment for laboratory tests.
Material supplies
– Access to medication for mental disorders. – Materials to provide care to children and adults. – Screening tool copies. – Paper.
Information technology
– Computers. – Internet platform. – Telephone lines. – Fax. – Copy machine. – Teleconferencing platform.

5 Collaborator aspirations

In order to develop a successful partnership, global mental health practitioners need to find a way to match the host's aspirations with that of collaborators.

Table A.16 Obtaining non-human resources

Low-cost strategies to obtain non-human resources
Key strategy Integrate mental health care into existing general health care services
General strategies to obtain non-human resources

- Conduct a needs and resources assessment before implementing the psychosocial care program to advocate for the allocation of specific funding to cover specific needs.
- Use existing resources within the health system that already have a pre-existing budget and modify them to fit the needs of the program.
- Charge patients a nominal fee for the mental health service.
- Use existing health programs for specific conditions other than mental disorders as platforms for providing psychosocial care (i.e. HIV).
- Choosing pilot programs as a strategy to obtain financial resources to establish a new program is a risky strategy to ensure sustainability.

➲ *Decision Point 1: Identifying collaborators*

Program planners can draw upon different types of collaborators, either in-country or foreign (Table A.17).

Table A.17 Identifying collaborators

Possible collaborators for scaling up

- Non-profit organizations related with health care provision academic institutions (either national or foreign).
- Public and private agencies interested in supporting the improvement of access to health.
- Professional societies of health professionals.
- Government institutions (either from the health sector or other).
- Retired or other mental health experts.
- Community or other grassroots organizations.
- Advocacy or consumer groups.

➲ *Decision Point 2: Identifying areas for collaboration*

Besides knowing who can collaborate with the host, it is important to identify what kinds of collaborations can most easily be pursued. Here are areas in which the collaborator assistance would be of greatest benefit for host communities (Table A.18).

6 Collaborator resources

Collaborators can best address the needs and aspirations of hosts by carefully establishing what resources are available for this collaboration.

Table A.18 Identifying areas for collaboration

Possible areas for collaboration
Financial
– Direct financial support via budget allocation or funding of a program component. – Establishment of private-public collaborations for funding and coordination of mental health programs. – Private companies can donate resources as part as social responsibility programs.
Technical
– Direct care provision by external mental health specialists. – On-site and remote training, support, and supervision. – Academic exchange programs (i.e. medical resident exchanges). – Addressing policy issues rather than only focusing on direct care provision. – Help local settings acquire, adapt, and implement pre-existing and new effective tools and mental health interventions, rather than developing new ones. – Extended on-site help on program development and implementation. – Non-profit organizations can oversee the administration of mental health programs at non-specialized level. – Capacity building, research, and policy development.
Material and program development
– Development of mental health awareness campaigns at a community level. – Development of short films locally to inform, educate, and raise awareness on mental disorders, using easy language in culturally relevant scenarios. – Facilitate access to library resources.

➲ *Decision Point: Identifying collaborator resources*

There are various financial, human, technical, and material resources that collaborators can bring to bear on global mental health collaborations (Table A.19).

7 Local liaison

According to the Wheel of Global Mental Health, a *local liaison* should be a person or organization that has a good understanding of the local burden of disease, health care system, human and other resources, infrastructure, culture, customs, language, politics, and history, as well as stigma towards mental illness.

➲ *Decision Point: Identifying the local liaison*

It is of course not possible to say exactly who would best serve as the local liaison in any given host community. However, we can anticipate the possible agencies that could function as hosts and as the source for a local liaison (Table A.20).

Table A.19 Identifying collaborator resources

Collaborator resources menu
Financial

– Funds: either one time grants or ongoing financial resources.

Human resources

– Remote and on-site specialized mental health manpower time and advice for:
  o care provision,
  o training, support, and supervision,
  o program design and implementation.
– Design and production of materials for care provision.

Technical and material

– Access to journals.
– Guidelines, books, and other technical resources for health providers.
– Provision of films, posters, or other types of displays to inform the population about mental health and psychiatric disorders.
– Supplies for care delivery.

Table A.20 Possible local liaison

Possible local liaison

– Government institutions linked to the health sector: at the national, regional, or community level.
– Non-governmental organizations.
– Professional associations related to the health sector.
– Academic institutions with health related programs.
– Consumer and advocacy groups.
– Community based organizations.

References

Carpio Barrantes, K. (2014) *A Model for Psychosocial Care Delivery: A Supplement for the Implementation of the mhGAP Program in Low-resource Settings.* (Master in Public Health Thesis), École des Hautes Études en Santé Publique (EHESP), France.

Eaton, J., McCay, L., Semrau, M., Chatterjee, S., Baingana, F., Araya, R., et al. (2011) 'Scale up of services for mental health in low-income and middle-income countries,' *The Lancet* vol. 378, no. 9802, pp. 1592–1603. doi: 10.1016/s0140-6736(11)60891-x.

IHME (2013) *The Global Burden of Disease: Generating Evidence, Guiding Policy* (European Union and European Free Trade Association Regional Edition), Institute for Health Metrics and Evaluation, Seattle, WA.

Lancet Global Mental Health Group, Chisholm, D., Flisher, A. J., Lund, C., Patel, V., Saxena, S., et al. (2007) 'Scale up services for mental disorders: a call for action,' *The Lancet* vol. 370, no. 9594, pp. 1241–1252. doi: 10.1016/S0140-6736(07)61242-2.

Samuels, D., Schuetz-Mueller, J., & Katz C.L. (2015) 'Disaster and global psychiatry,' in: W. Goodman, A. Simon, & A. New, *Mount Sinai Expert Guide: Psychiatry*, Wiley and Sons, New Jersey. In press.

Whiteford, H. A. & Baxter, A. J. (2013) 'The Global Burden of Disease 2010 Study: what does it tell us about mental disorders in Latin America?' *Revista Brasileira De Psiquiatria* vol. 35, no. 2, pp. 111–112. doi: 10.1590/1516-4446-2012-3502.

WHO (2001) *Mental Health: A Call for Action by World Health Ministers*. Paper presented at the World Health Assembly, Geneva.

WHO (2008) *mhGAP: Mental Health Gap Action Programme: Scaling Up Care for Mental, Neurological and Substance Use Disorders* (ed. T. Satyanand), World Health Organization, France.

WHO (2010) *mhGAP Intervention Guide for Mental, Neurological and Substance Use Disorders in Non-specialized Health Settings: Mental Health Gap Action Programme (mhGAP)*, World Health Organization, Italy.

Index